We Learned to

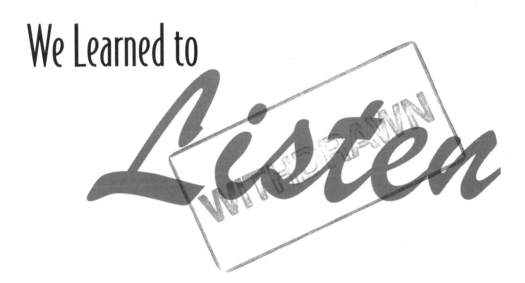

D1638165

en Estabrooks

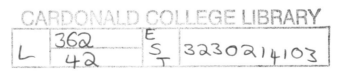
ALEXANDER GRAHAM BELL ASSOCIATION FOR THE DEAF AND HARD OF HEARING • 3417 VOLTA PLACE, NW, WASHINGTON, DC 20007

Library of Congress Control Number: 2005920597

ISBN 0-88200-222-8

The Alexander Graham Bell Association for the Deaf and Hard of Hearing (AG Bell) is a lifelong resource, support network, and advocate for listening, learning, talking, and living independently with hearing loss. Through publications, outreach training, scholarships, and financial aid, AG Bell promotes the use of spoken language and hearing technology. Headquartered in Washington, DC, with chapters located in the United States and Canada and a network of international affiliates, AG Bell's global presence provides its members and the public with the support they need — close to home. With over a century of service, AG Bell supports its mission: Advocating Independence through Listening and Talking! For more information, contact AG Bell at (202) 337-5220 or visit the AG Bell website at www.agbell.org.

Alexander Graham Bell Association for the Deaf and Hard of Hearing, Inc.
3417 Volta Place, NW
Washington, DC 20007–2778, USA
www.agbell.org

Cover design: Kathleen Carbonetti
Editing, text design & formatting: Christopher Howland

Printed in the United States
10 9 8 7 6 5 4 3 2 1

Contents

WE LEARNED TO LISTEN IS DEDICATED TO THE PARENTS AND FAMILIES OF THOSE WHO share their stories within these pages and to the professionals who were fortunate to be part of their lives.

Preface

WE LEARNED TO LISTEN IS A COURAGEOUS WORK ABOUT A GROUP OF TRUE PIONEERS.

It is about the lives of nine individuals who are deaf who grew up during a time when hearing technology was very limited. There were no digital hearing aids and no cochlear implants. But these individuals defied what many people expected would happen. They learned to listen. They learned to speak.

In the high-tech world of the 21st century, there are greater opportunities than ever for children who are born deaf or hard of hearing, or who acquire deafness in early childhood . . . opportunities to learn to hear, to listen, to converse in spoken language, to go to school with their peers, and to lead bountiful lives with abundant choices . . . choices that most of us take for granted.

We Learned to Listen was written to encourage parents and professionals who work in partnership with these children and to inspire any reader who is fascinated by lives of resilience.

We Learned to Listen is a celebration, and ultimately is a gift of love.

Warren Estabrooks
Toronto, Canada
Spring 2005

Acknowledgments

WE LEARNED TO LISTEN WAS CREATED BY AN OUTSTANDING COLLABORATIVE EFFORT OVER a period of three years. My heartfelt thanks go to:

- My contributing authors — Jonathan Samson, Karen MacIver-Lux, John-David Humphreys, Nora McKellin, Richard Farr, Vanessa Vaughan, Sol Fried, Frances Mezei, and Ellen Rhoades — for sharing their lives openly, honestly, and lovingly to bring the dream of this project to life;

- The staff and Board of Directors of the Alexander Graham Bell Association for the Deaf and Hard of Hearing, for their support of publications of all auditory and oral options for children and adults with hearing loss;

- Dale Atkins, my friend, for enthusiastically embracing this project and writing her attentive, insightful foreword;

- Chris Howland, my copy editor, for his diligence, professionalism, care, and attention to detail;

- John Craig and Ariella Samson, for their continued mentorship, support, and love;

- The staff of the Auditory Learning Centre of the Learning to Listen Foundation (my angels: Karen, Lisa, and Mila), for their love, understanding, respect, loyalty, and dedication;

- Mary Woodburn, a very special secretary; and

- Pierre-Roch Côté, Michelle Benjamin, Laurie Monsebraaten, and Jeff Keay, my enthusiastic proofreaders.

WIE

Foreword BY DALE ATKINS, Ph.D.

WE LEARNED TO LISTEN IS AN INSPIRING COLLECTION OF PERSONAL STORIES BY A UNIQUE group of individuals who are deaf — individuals who continue to bravely face, and even defy, many people's perceptions of who they are and what they should be. In this wonderful book, we follow as each author travels from a daunting world of silence to one in which he or she has become an integral part of a "hearing" society. We witness the exceptional drive, will, and sense of self that has made each of these author's lives so remarkable. It is rare when a reader can be privy to such private, sometimes joyous, sometimes angst-ridden, thoughts and feelings.

Different parents have different goals for their children, and the methods of achieving these goals may be very diverse, especially if a child is deaf or hard of hearing. With little knowledge of deafness and its many conflicting points of view, it is challenging to make sound educational, linguistic, psychosocial, technological, and even medical decisions for the child. Parents need to follow their own beliefs about what is best not only for their child but also their own family system.

We all want to be the best parents possible and give our children the greatest opportunities in life. Often when we are most vulnerable, we are required to make decisions for them that will affect their future. Every juncture in our children's lives is burdened with the gnawing question, "Is this the right decision?" We invest ourselves fully with the faith and trust that our children will flourish along the route we have determined for them, and ultimately along the route they will choose for themselves as they try to reach their greatest social, academic, and spiritual potential.

In *We Learned to Listen*, we experience the anguish, fear, and loneliness that have accompanied these nine individuals throughout their diverse lives. But we also celebrate their strength, courage, determination, resilience, and triumphs.

We Learned to Listen is a rare treat indeed.

Dr. Atkins is a psychologist, author, and television personality with a private practice in New York City.

CHAPTER 1

Jonathan

Jonathan Samson

"YOUR SON HAS A PROFOUND HEARING LOSS."

As I stood in the sound booth with my wife, my infant son, and the audiologist, I thought of how my parents must have felt when they heard a similar statement about me some 30 years earlier — that overwhelming, earth-shaking moment which would forever change their lives.

I began to reflect on the various stages and unique moments of my life. Even though the successes and failures I have experienced were my own, it was the guidance, encouragement, and assistance of a large network of people that inspired me to constantly move forward despite being deaf. This network of my parents, family, and many talented professionals gave me the tools and taught me vital lessons in adapting to my hearing loss.

I am reminded of the old Chinese proverb: *Give a man a fish and you feed him for a day. Teach a man to fish and you feed him for a lifetime.* That is what my parents did for me, and my wife and I will do the same for our son Jacob.

Suspicions Confirmed

I was born three weeks early, on a Saturday in May of 1971, spoiling a country picnic my parents had planned that day with friends. Other than my early arrival, however, there was nothing unusual about my birth. Unaware of the difficult road that lay ahead, my parents simply enjoyed the euphoria of their first-born child and basked in the wishes and congratulations that came from family and friends throughout the world. The excitement included visits from both sets of grandparents, arriving in Toronto from afar to see their new grandson. Their visits culminated in the Jewish ritual of Brit Milah one week later, after which my parents settled down to start their new family life.

Almost immediately, my mother suspected that something might be wrong. In my new nursery, which was being transformed from a sewing room, the ironing board crashed to the floor one day, startling my mother. I just smiled obliviously, undisturbed. My mother said she chose to look past this incident since she wasn't ready to have her dreams and excitement crushed. It was several months before she revealed her fears to my father, who admitted that he also was worried I might be deaf. Although my father said he wasn't ready to discuss the issue, my parents did decide to say something to my pediatrician. The pediatrician, however, convinced them they were being a bit neurotic and overanxious.

It wasn't easy for my parents that, at this time, their friends' children were responding normally to sounds and speech, some having even reached the point of babbling. I, on the other hand, remained focused on play and paid attention to nothing else.

At 11 months of age, my profound hearing loss was finally confirmed, though surprisingly the news was announced to my parents in a hospital hallway, where they were left to fend for themselves. No additional information or materials were provided, but at least the audiologist made earmold impressions for hearing aids and booked me for a return appointment. Despite the devastating news, my parents felt some relief knowing the problem had been identified as deafness and not a cognitive impairment.

My parents immediately went to the nearby university library to do research. They also visited schools for children who are deaf or hard of hearing and were appalled at the low academic levels and low expectations in those schools. During their research, they discovered the importance of "residual hearing" in remediating deafness. They found that if the residual hearing of a child with hearing loss is properly exploited through excellent amplification technology, he or she can learn to listen and talk. Armed with this knowledge, my parents decided that would be the path they would follow for me.

Therapy Begins

I was fitted with two body-worn hearing aids at 11 months and, about a month later, began auditory training sessions with Louise Crawford at the Hospital for Sick Children in Toronto. This was the start of my journey through the Auditory-Verbal world. Miss Crawford was one of the pioneers of the Auditory-Verbal movement in Canada in the 1960s and '70s. Following the teachings of Daniel Ling, Doreen Pollack, and Helen Beebe, she carried the torch for A-V therapy in her immediate hometown of Toronto. To this day, Louise Crawford maintains a great love for children who are deaf or hard of hearing. Her former students hold her in high regard and have tremendous gratitude for what she did for us and our parents. Her teaching style was quite formal, quite structured, and actually quite perfect for a troublemaker like me.

My mother became my teacher. Every day, she spent hours pointing out sounds, providing structured lessons, and expanding language during my playtime. She would often crawl on the floor with me guiding my introduction to sound awareness. It was a big commitment to spend the majority of the day bathing me in those sounds, working on my language development through play, or sitting at the kitchen table for formal lessons. My father would reinforce everything on which my mother worked and helped with my siblings so I could have the attention I needed to succeed.

I would visit Miss Crawford once a week and am told that I constantly embarrassed my mother with my misbehavior. Miss Crawford's rule was when a child misbehaved, it was the parent who had to leave the room. Thus, everyone who walked down that hospital corridor knew that it was Mrs. Samson's child who was not being a good boy.

I do not recall my early lessons. I remember the drive downtown to the hospital, the playroom, and the coloring books in the waiting area. Yet, my memory of stepping into the lessons is blocked. Despite constant worries that I was not making much progress, the hard work paid off. Many parents and professionals ask me today how I talk so well with such a profound hearing loss. When they do, it is a compliment that honors my parents' hard work, dedication, commitment, and tremendous patience.

I spent $7\frac{1}{2}$ years with Miss Crawford before I "graduated"; however, my parents felt it wouldn't hurt to keep working on my speech and listening development. I began sessions with Warren Estabrooks, who at the time was teaching at the Metro Toronto School for the Deaf. He taught me after school in what used to be a storage room, the only available space we could find. Warren later relocated to North York General Hospital, where we had a much nicer room filled with toys to stimulate and motivate learning. We spent many years working together, and I remember enjoying that time filled with listening, speech, and songs. The songs were my favorite part, especially when Warren played his guitar.

Music, rhythm, and rhyme were integral parts of my therapy. Emphasis was also placed on speech practice, such as "baa baa baa," "boo boo boo," and "bee bee bee." And, to help with speech and intonation, we tried our hand at tongue twisters.

My mother attended the lessons with Warren, which is a requirement of Auditory-Verbal therapy. However, when I was about 13 years old, she stopped coming because I was too old to be accompanied. I would bring the work home, though, and we would still practice together daily. Throughout the lessons, Warren would weave together humor, sarcasm, songs, and conversational skills. Those lessons were critical in developing my good sense of humor.

I have been fortunate to have had such special teachers in my life. These teachers recognized my strengths, encouraged me, and helped develop my potential to be successful. I continue to have good relationships with them. I hold them in high regard and will always be grateful for what they have done for me and my parents. I wouldn't have obtained such personal success if it weren't for Miss Crawford and Warren.

Time for School

My early years were fairly normal in a reckless sort of way. My mother described me as a very hyper child who was typically loud, unruly, and always misbehaving. She said she didn't dare take me out in public places because I would throw temper tantrums. Surprisingly, I was fairly good when visiting other people, and I was always good with adults.

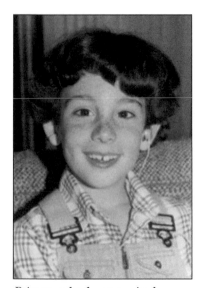

Primary school was a mixed experience for me. There were difficult times in which episodes of intolerance affected me.

Until I started school at age 2½, I spent all day in lessons with my mother in both formal and informal settings. Even bath time was spent in "therapy." My mother had contacted Daniel Ling shortly after my hearing loss was diagnosed, driving to Montreal at one point to meet with him personally, and she had kept in touch with him. One of his earliest pieces of advice was for her to use an ear horn to communicate with me while I was bathing, since he felt I still had enough residual hearing for it to be beneficial. Because of that, it seemed my mother was always within a foot of me.

As I got older, I became involved in various extracurricular activities such as Cub Scouts, Boy Scouts, swimming, skating, soccer, skiing, and Hebrew lessons. I even took piano lessons for more than 10 years. Also, as an avid reader, I would go to the library every week to bring home the latest books.

When it was time to go to kindergarten, my parents tried to enroll me in the local school, only to have the principal flatly refuse to accept me. He felt it was inappropriate for a child with hearing loss to attend his school and the law at the time supported his decision. Despite various pleas by my parents to his better nature, he stood his ground, so my parents had no choice but to look elsewhere. Fortunately, they found a private school in Toronto that was willing to take me.

I have a positive recollection of my two short years at Bayview Glen. The teachers, for one, were very accommodating. Although there were no support services available in the school, my parents actually didn't want me to have any at that stage. They simply wanted me to enjoy being a child, enjoy socialization, learn to play, and just be with other children. Ultimately, the principal at the local school left before I was supposed to start first grade and the incoming principal made a policy switch and allowed me to enroll.

On my first day of elementary school, I received a rude awakening to the reality of how some children can act. Until then, most kids I met generally were good to me, since at the age of 4 no one really cares whether you wear hearing aids or speak in an unusual manner. But that first day in first grade, while sitting at a table with several other kids, we were told by the teacher to introduce ourselves. The girl next to me had already stated her name. Perhaps for clarification or some other reason, I asked her to repeat it: *Stacey*. I repeated it and it probably came out as "a-e." The girl laughed at me and mimicked my pronunciation, and shortly thereafter all the kids at the table did the same. I recall not being sure what to make of their reaction, but I don't remember what I did next. I just remember the incident.

Not too long after that, my mother made a presentation to the class to explain what hearing loss was all about and how hearing aids work. I recall all the kids listening through a stethoscope attached to a hearing aid. In some ways, this presentation helped the kids understand me better, but it also drew further attention to me and gave the bullies some ammunition. To be fair, they probably would have figured it out quickly for themselves.

For many years, I tolerated people talking to me from behind or with their mouths covered or clenched. However, the presentation about deafness was beneficial because it created better awareness and more tolerance, which eventually helped break down barriers and misconceptions. Social relationships tend to get better when people become aware of the implications of living with a hearing loss. Even if only one person changes because of such a presentation, then it is a success.

Primary school proved to be a mixed experience for me. Although my childhood was generally a happy one, there were difficult times in which certain episodes of intolerance affected my outlook and attitude. I didn't really have any close friends in school during this period. At best, most kids were acquaintances who seemed more interested in the treehouse in our yards or the latest toys I had. This latter point revealed the true hypocrisy of the bullies at school. They would pick on me during the day and then play at my house after school. My so-called "friends" would make fun of me in front of their own friends. Therefore, I became friendly with others who were being picked on, which in turn made the bullies hold me in contempt for being friendly to them. I learned a lot about human nature without really knowing it.

My family was extremely supportive and gave me a comfort zone. Some of my school friends treated me well on a one-to-one basis. In fact, one classmate who was popular gave me enormous protection and shelter. I learned to pick my battles and that there was a way around or through every situation. I learned instinctively not to take these things too personally. As much as I disliked being picked on, it was really just a short moment in time. At the end of the day, I was able to realize that I was a person first and that my deafness was secondary. My parents gave me excellent tools for being confident and staying positive.

A Normal Family

Throughout my childhood, my family provided me a sense of normalcy. I never asked why I was deaf or said, "Why me?" When my younger sister was born, however, my mother recalls that I said I wanted her to be hearing impaired as well. That shocked my mother, but I told her it was so I wouldn't be alone. This, my mother said, was a sign that I didn't view deafness negatively, but rather as something to share.

My parents instilled confidence in me early by helping me integrate listening into my communication and social skills. We followed developmental patterns of listening, language, and cognition to stimulate natural communication, which is a principle of Auditory-Verbal therapy. For example, when we went out, especially to restaurants, most people couldn't understand me. Naturally, they would look at my parents for an explanation. My parents would direct them back to me so I could speak for myself. I quickly learned that I could do what anybody else could do.

My parents firmly believed in equality among their children, but that was easier said than done. They had to give more attention to me than my brother,

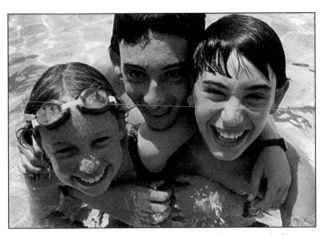

While my mother spent countless hours with me, my father gave my younger siblings Noam and Alana the attention they needed. My parents also created special trips for them alone.

Noam, and my sister, Alana, both of whom had normal hearing. Therefore, while my mother spent countless hours with me, my father gave my younger siblings the attention they needed. My parents also created special opportunities for them by taking them out on trips alone. Consequently, I believe their actions guided my siblings and me to the dynamic relationship we have today. However, it was not always that way. Like most brothers and sisters, we fought like cats and dogs one minute and played with our G.I. Joes the next. We drove our parents mad.

Although my mother did the bulk of the work with me, my father's main role was to support her. He tried to make things easier for her by carrying out daily routines and errands. He was also responsible for giving us our baths, driving us to programs, and doing story time each night.

As I got older and started to use the telephone, I developed a system where I had someone interpret orally for me. This worked by having two phones in the same location. I would lipread the "interpreter" who was listening on one phone and then respond into mine, and the conversation would flow naturally with little or no delay. (The poor family member who had the good fortune to answer the phone would often be trapped into this role.) When I needed to make a call, I would grab someone — anyone — regardless of what they were doing. This often led to heated discussions, so my parents laid down firm ground rules. My siblings could not trade their role in this for another chore, nor could they hold me hostage by withholding their services. In return, I had to try to wait until the sibling was finished with his or her TV program or game. This was somewhat unsuccessful. Eventually, when I reached the "dating stage," my sister just loved helping me out because it provided her the latest gossip. At that point, I learned to use the TTY and relay service to protect my privacy.

I must have driven my brother to insanity in the days before closed captioning. Every minute of television watching was spent with me asking, "What did they say?" And, though I was supposed to wait until the commercials to ask, I usually couldn't. Between the TV, telephone, fights, and the inability to share, it is amazing that Noam and I not only have a good sibling relationship today, but also work together in the family business.

My extended family was always very supportive of my parents and me, but they all lived out of town. I was very close with my grandparents. I only saw my paternal grandparents about once a year on special trips. My mother's parents lived outside of Toronto and I would see them during the summer and during school holidays, as well as a few other times throughout the year. When my maternal grandmother was in town, she would attend my Auditory-Verbal lessons and would make a conscientious effort to incorporate those lessons when interacting with me. Her native tongue was Hungarian and she usually spoke with my mother in that language. Whenever I came into the room, they would always make an effort to switch to English, which wasn't easy for her. However, she knew that no matter how difficult it was, it was more important that I follow the conversation. Years later, she would come to live with us when she was sick with cancer and surgery had caused her to lose the use of her vocal cords. The irony was that I became her interpreter by reading her lips and telling people what she had said.

Valuable Assistance

During my primary school years, I had several itinerant teachers who took me out of class 2–3 times a week. I spent a lot of time working with them on research and presentation skills, organizing homework, and concentrating on my weak subjects. We also did extra auditory skills work and played games to enhance my language and speech development. When I was about 9, I started telephone training, working on basic skills such as learning how to recognize a dial tone, a busy signal, and the presence of a voice. I learned to understand commonly used names, phrases, days of the week, and numbers. I also developed strategies to understand a message by using keywords for each letter of the alphabet.

We also spent time developing practical classroom strategies and troubleshooting the FM system that I used in class. Much to my teachers' dismay, the system constantly broke down or would be uncharged. My teachers and parents were convinced that I was trying to sabotage it — after all, the system was bulky and looked like a neon sign strapped to my chest. Once, the principal hauled me into his office and reprimanded me.

Nevertheless, when the FM system did work, my teachers would quite often forget to switch the transmitter off while talking to the principal, disciplining a child, or going to the bathroom. My classmates could hear everything coming through my leaky earmolds. It's a shame I could never understand what they were hearing and, thus, laughing about. It didn't really matter, though, because those were my very popular moments. By the time I reached high school, I had won the war against the FM system and managed without it from then on. In later years, well after I graduated from university, I came to realize its advantages. Today's technology has progressed so far that the FM components are now built into the hearing aid or come as a snap-on to the aid or cochlear implant. That is a far cry from the big box-size unit I wore in the early days.

Ultimately, the itinerant teachers were my source of support, someone to whom I could turn to discuss my troubles at school or for just a little bit of extra help. They were my advance team, usually showing up at my school before the term began to talk with my regular teachers about my needs. They helped smooth out any bumps in the road as I passed through public school. They were also my encouragement to learn to advocate on my own and to try to problem-solve before coming to them. By the time I reached high school, I had honed the skills required for living and learning independently even beyond high school.

I also learned about my ticket to free rides. I disliked gym so much that I instructed a naive teacher that deafness and physical education did not go hand in hand, so she let me out of the class. This wonderful arrangement didn't last long because my mother happened to visit the school one day early in the year, right during gym period. She exposed me.

There were many teachers (and, of course, substitute teachers) who fell for my stories over the years. I turned a disadvantage — my hearing loss — into an advantage.

Big Adjustment

When I moved on to junior high, it was a big adjustment. Although most of my classmates from elementary school came with me, I was now surrounded by many more kids and faced a complete change of structure. I was no longer in one classroom all day. I had to go to several and needed to adapt to a lot of new kids and several different teachers. However, I was armed with much more ammunition than before, some in my control and some not.

The junior high years are a time of social exploration for most kids. In my case, the boys suddenly were interested only in girls, which meant my former tormenters ignored me as they spent their energies elsewhere. The girls were not kind to me either, and the pretty ones had no qualms showing what they thought of me. By this time, however, I was immune to their efforts, given that I had been through this for some time. My social development was delayed compared to my peers, and my interest in girls wasn't as great as the other boys. Besides, their actions toward me didn't help my interest at all.

Furthermore, I was a good student, with a reputation for finishing my assignments on time and earning high marks. All of a sudden, most of my peers became very interested in my homework. They would either ask to copy my work or to be my study or group work partner — a far cry from being picked last for everything in elementary school. I was able to use my new popularity to preserve the peace and make it through junior high.

When I started junior high, I spent many lunch hours in the computer room, usually playing games. Then one day I discovered baseball and other sports and moved away from the computer and onto the field. That helped me interact more with other kids and gave me some measure of respect.

My classes were more difficult since they required much more concentration and a variety of strategies (i.e., sitting close to the front of the room, pre-reading the work for class, discussing the material with the teacher, and looking at my classmates' notes). These were tools of survival, and important skills to hone for high school. They also helped me overcome the extra challenges presented by my hearing loss. My classmates' notes were not, by themselves, particularly useful, but they did guide me in knowing what was going on in class and provided some context. Subsequently, my teachers would confirm, clarify, and fill in the gaps, either after class or after school. Advocating for myself helped me stay on top of things.

I continued to have the support of an itinerant teacher once a week, but her role changed to spending more time on my language rather than speech. She helped me with my various regular teachers to ensure that my needs were met. The itinerant teacher had to convey the importance of using the FM system, good seating position, and, more crucially, patience and tolerance. A positive attitude by my teachers would set a good example for my classmates and create an atmosphere where I could feel comfortable and succeed. So if the teacher didn't understand what I said or needed to repeat something for me, her patience would set the tone for others in the class.

When I turned 13, I was required to be called up to the Torah in Synagogue and read from it in Hebrew. My Bar Mitzvah was a monumental occasion. I had prepared for nearly a year. In front of family, friends, and teachers, I proudly read a portion of the Torah Scroll in Hebrew. In my religion, this meant that I had moved symbolically from boyhood to manhood. I also had done something my parents never thought or imagined I would do when I was first diagnosed with hearing loss. It was indeed an accomplishment I will never forget.

A Time of Self-Initiative

In high school, I was no longer subjected to the daily ridicule I had faced in elementary school. I had entered a much bigger world of students and teachers and I felt free of many of the constraints placed on me by former classmates. It was also a time of self-initiative.

I was allowed to help in choosing which high school I wanted to attend. There were two public schools near my house and I visited both with my parents. One was large and operated on a term schedule, meaning you took the same eight subjects all year. I decided to go the other school. It was much smaller and operated on a semester schedule. You took four subjects one semester and four the next.

At this stage of my life, I began to take more responsibility for myself. I made sure I discussed important issues with my teachers, such as having them face the class and not the blackboard when they spoke and ensuring that I understood when they announced exams or papers. I began to advocate for myself to ensure that my own needs would be met. I had more control of the courses I wanted and needed. For instance, one of the requirements for graduation was three years of French, a subject I disliked immensely. I discovered a loophole involving hearing loss and language that allowed me to obtain an exemption. I made an agreement with the principal to substitute French for a music class and three years of Latin. I excelled in both subjects and became a peer tutor. I honestly don't think he ever noticed the irony and discrepancy in this swap.

I quickly made my mark in high school by becoming involved in as many activities as possible. I worked in the library and was on the student council. With a greater mixture of people with whom to interact, and with greater freedom, I made friends. I didn't belong to a specific group, but I was on friendly terms with several groups of people. This would actually help me later when I campaigned for high school president.

I was friendly with several girls at this time, and I was content to leave it at that level instead of dating. By 11th grade, however, I began to get more involved socially, and when my social calendar got busier, my grades went down.

My crowning achievement in high school was being elected student council president. This, I felt, was the ultimate acceptance and a huge stepping stone for me. I ran a hard campaign against a very popular student. I think the shockwave that went through the school after my victory was more one of admiration than amazement. I ran on the slogan:

> *I may be deaf,*
> *But you're not blind,*
> *So when it's time to vote,*
> *Keep me in mind.*

I wanted people to understand that if I am comfortable with whom I am, they should be, too. In my speeches, I encouraged people to look past my hearing loss and did my best to assure them it wouldn't be a factor as president. And, like any politician, I promised them lots of dance parties, social events, and sports. It was a defining moment in my social development.

My itinerant support was reduced to once every three weeks, and I spent most of that time on grammar and presentation skills. I made the choice to no longer use an FM system; therefore, I had to work much harder to keep up with my classes and school work. That meant regularly communicating with my teachers, as well as my classmates, to fill in gaps. I also sat at the front of the classroom. In one geography course, my teacher heavily favored audio-visual equipment and often taught the class from the back of a darkened room with the slide projector on. This put me at a distinct disadvantage, but the teacher and I were able to work out a plan that included tutoring from an older geography student.

My after-school time was spent volunteering for a local seniors group, which involved going to their homes and helping with housework, errands, gardening, and shoveling snow in the winter. Since I had an entrepreneurial streak in me, I also started my own greeting card business and donated some of the proceeds to local charities. In my last year of high school, I organized a dance marathon for leukemia research and also coordinated the senior prom.

I graduated with honors and was named my school's Student of the Year at the graduation ceremony, with my parents and my regular and itinerant teachers (a great team) in attendance. I prepared to make a big jump into a much bigger world, with much less support and guidance: university.

An Active Social Life

Since I felt it was time for me to spread my wings, I decided to go the University of Western Ontario in London, about a 2-hour drive from Toronto. As an Auditory-Verbal graduate, I was a veteran of self-advocacy and felt confident and independent enough to strike out on my own. I followed the same strategies in university that I had in high school, both in class and socially. I had the benefit of additional tools, however, such as the use of a notetaker in my classes. What I wasn't prepared for, was that I needed to start from scratch from a social standpoint (since I was the only one from my high school to go to that university). Initially, I received notice from university officials that I hadn't qualified for on-campus residency and would have to arrange for accommodations on my own. I felt strongly that to avoid isolation and get a head start on expanding my social connections, I had to make it into on-campus residence somehow. I secured letters on my behalf from various sources — including from Dr. Ling, who happened to be the dean of one of the faculties — and submitted them to the registrar asking for reconsideration. The registrar agreed and I was given my own room, which had built-in wiring for the fire alarm.

My first night went well, I thought. I slept nicely, but was awakened about 6:45 a.m. to extremely loud banging on my door which caused my bed to thump up and down. My floormates were using a metal trash can against the door hoping the loud noise would somehow wake me up. (I slept without my hearing aids on.) I was informed that the residents were being called downstairs to the auditorium for a meeting with the building manager at 7. I got dressed hastily and made my way downstairs, unsure of what the whole commotion was about. After all of the residents (some 1,250 of them.) settled down, the building manager came into the room and angrily proceeded to lecture us on the dangers of false fire alarms. As he brought in the captain of the local firehouse to talk to us, I turned to the person next to me and asked why he was discussing this issue, especially so early in the morning. He turned to me a little bleary eyed and informed me that someone had pulled the alarm at 2 a.m., forcing evacuation of the entire building for more than an hour until the fire department could clear the scene. I looked in amazement and realized that I had slept through the whole commotion since the building manager had forgotten to switch on the flashing light in my room.

Living away from home and going to a university where I didn't know anyone was very difficult in the beginning. After a few weeks, however, I met Steve Dalal, an older student who became a good friend and helped my transition. He was the first of several very good and special university friends with whom I still have close bonds today. They were able to recognize my abilities and accepted me for who I was. They seemed oblivious to my hearing loss and would treat me like anyone else.

Classes were unlike high school. They were much larger and configured differently. It was not so simple to sit at the front of the class because some professors often walked or moved about the room. Therefore, I had to learn each professor's quirks and habits and position myself accordingly. Although I spoke with all of my professors beforehand, and most of them were accommodating, I did have one who barked at me, "Tough, that's the way it is." I had notetakers for all my classes and, when possible, I would try to obtain a copy of the professor's lecture notes. When necessary, I made use of the professor's

> I felt strongly that to avoid isolation and get a head start on expanding my social connections, I had to make it into on-campus residence.

office hours to go over the notes from the class to ensure that I didn't miss out on too much.

My social life became very active during my four years at Western Ontario. Having access to more people in residence, as well as being involved with various clubs and the student council, kept me from feeling isolated and promoted my social skills. I spent many a weekend or evening at a local bar or attending one of numerous parties in the area. It was important to have fun.

I got involved with the student council again, and became vice president of finance my final year, responsible for a budget of $11 million. That was another tight election for me, with several obstacles and challenges to overcome. I won by a single vote.

I graduated with a B.A. in political science, and was singled out for personal congratulations by the university president during convocation.

Proving Myself in the Working World

As an undergraduate, I worked during the summer for a money management firm in downtown Toronto. After graduation, I went to work in a bank doing customer relations. My relationships with colleagues and bosses were mostly good, but I always had to fight to prove myself, especially when working for clients who were not used to my disability. Once a customer came into the bank and, not seeing the sign in front of me that indicated I had a hearing loss, proceeded to ask for a sum of money, the amount of which I could not understand because of his heavy accent. After repeating himself several times, he finally screamed at me, "Are you deaf or something?" I responded in the affirmative and guided his attention to the sign in front of me, which only seemed to anger him more. He yelled again, "Why the hell don't you wear hearing aids?" Another affirmative response gained me a scowl. After writing his request down and leaving the bank, my colleagues and I doubled over in laughter at this whole comical scene. A few hours later, a woman came in, saw the sign, appeared at my desk, and proceeded to inform me over the course of 10 or 15 minutes why she had so much difficulty hearing and how people didn't help her enough. Then, in mid-sentence, she stopped. Realization dawned on her. She looked at me and said, "Oh, this sign is for *you*? I thought this was a line for the hearing impaired."

I left the bank after a short time since I felt the people there didn't recognize my potential. I believed the bank was using my hearing loss to portray itself as an equal opportunity employer. I consequently went into the family business of investments, where I still work today with my father and brother. My job allows me the flexibility to work at giving back to the community as a role model and a board member of various organizations.

Friends for Life

Since I was always mainstreamed, my friends typically had normal hearing and came either from the schools I attended or from my local neighborhood. During my childhood, I had three close friends, two with normal hearing. One was a neighbor and the other was the son of my mother's good friend. The third was John Humphreys, who like me had a profound hearing loss. The two of us created our own support network, and through our friendship we developed and perfected strategies. The focus of our relationship was not on our impairments; rather, it was on a set of interests and values. We had sleepovers, or met downtown to go to movies or to the mall. My parents allowed me, after several practice runs, to take the subway downtown on my own. They gave me two quarters: one to call them once I reached my destination so they knew I was safe; the other to call before I came home. John and I would flag someone down in the middle of the shopping mall or go into a store and explain that we were deaf and had to call home. We asked if they would be kind enough to call for us. Then we would take the 50 cents and buy some ice cream. After doing this a few times, however, my parents caught on. We were disciplined and forced to donate the money to charity.

This was the basis of many of our exploits. John taught me a lot about true friendship by unconditionally accepting me.

Friends have come and gone, but people like John and Steve Dalal always remained close to me. Our friendships were clear-cut. They were based on a set of common interests and goals and had nothing to do with hearing loss. That just wasn't an issue and, therefore, something I cherish highly. Over the years, with the exception of John, I didn't make friends in the world of the deaf and hard of hearing, nor did I actively participate in events related to that world. Although I attended conferences and sat on many panels that discussed the issue of deafness, it was always from an emotionally detached viewpoint, after which I would return home to my hearing world.

Sadly, I actually looked down on others who were deaf but didn't speak or listen. It took me many years to get over this attitude. When I finally did, I started to make other friends whom I value today. One is Tania, the woman who would become my wife, and another is Karen MacIver-Lux. I met Karen when she applied for a job at the Learning to Listen Foundation (LTLF). Karen, her husband Martin and I quickly became close friends. We found our backgrounds very similar and shared a lot of experiences as a result. The year I met them was the year I received my cochlear implant. Karen became a big part of my rehabilitation by practicing daily with me on the telephone. Her patience with me was a blessing and, without a doubt, the strongest reason I can use the telephone today with relative ease and comfort.

Finding the Girl of my Dreams

As a university student, I started dating. In fact, it was easier for me to date during that period (rather than after I graduated) since people knew me and my hearing loss was generally not an issue. When I dated after graduating, my deafness either surprised my dates or created uncertainty for them. I always made sure my dates knew in advance, and they all indicated it wasn't an issue, although I'm sure it was. Ironically, I was the one who discriminated. I refused to date women with a hearing loss. Once, a friend of my mother wanted to set me up on a date and I refused, explaining that it was "double the trouble." My mother lightly smacked the back of my head in disbelief.

I always wanted to date and eventually marry a person with normal hearing. This, I felt, was important as a way of acceptance. Over the years, I realized what a ridiculous notion that was and ultimately agreed to go out with a woman who had a similar hearing loss. Nothing came of it. About that time, I also went out with someone who lived about 40 minutes away, which I thought was too far to travel for a relationship. (The date in my mind was over before I even met the girl.) Strangely enough, a month later, I met Tania at the Alexander Graham Bell Association for the Deaf and Hard of Hearing convention in Little Rock, Arkansas. Tania captured my interest, and despite the fact that she lived in London, England, we communicated through e-mails and online chat rooms, eventually traveling back and forth between our countries for nearly two years before getting married.

The real advantage in the end was the commonality we shared and the belief that we didn't need to explain ourselves. Tania has had similar experiences, coming from an auditory background, studying away from home, and being able to advocate strongly for herself. When I met her, I noted that she was a wonderful person, with a very social and bubbly personality who had friends all over the world. Today, she is very accomplished, with a master's degree in educational and school psychology, and a teaching degree in primary school education. She also is a teacher of the deaf, dedicated to helping children reach their potential by drawing upon her own experiences and working with supportive parents. We both knew the obstacles with which we had struggled, and we focused our relationship on everything else but deafness. Our wedding in London, a beautiful and moving moment in our lives, was attended by many of our greatest friends and supporters. We settled in Toronto and a new chapter began for both of us.

Benefiting from Technology

I have found that the key to a successful relationship or marriage is understanding, mutual respect, and good communication. The first two have come easily for us because of our similar backgrounds, although our personalities are quite different. Our communication, however, has its ups and downs. Calling through the house to the other is often a one-way dead end, and arguments between two deaf people who know all the tricks of the trade (i.e., closing one's eyes when you don't want to lipread the other, etc.) makes for a bumpy ride (also known as a "normal" relationship). However, Tania and I have built a strong foundation by supporting and motivating one another. We both know that our successes cannot be accomplished alone — that it takes teamwork.

Modern technology is our best friend. Tania and I have taken advantage of many devices to make our lives as easy and comfortable as possible. We both have two-way interactive "pagers" (i.e., Blackberries) to communicate in lieu of a cell phone. Our house is wired with flashing lights for doorbells, alarms, and smoke detection systems. Our front door has a video camera so we can see who is there. We have "call display" on our telephones to see who is calling before answering. We use the computer and a video camera (a combination of typing, speaking through microphones, and listening via the computer speakers) to communicate with Tania's parents in England, as well as many other friends throughout the world. And, closed captioning on our televisions makes shows and movies a pleasure to watch. These devices are complementary to our listening skills. Listening was difficult with our hearing aids, but now that we both have cochlear implants, sounds and speech have become much more meaningful.

A Door Opens

Getting a cochlear implant was a difficult decision, just like any type of surgery. A well-respected audiologist cautioned me that long-term use of my powerful linear hearing aids would likely destroy the remainder of my residual hearing over time. He suggested I look into getting an implant, and after talking with many professionals, teachers, and implant users, I saw this as another technological wonder that would make my life much easier and better. So, in August 1997, I underwent implant surgery and received my processor a month later. At the end of September, a few days before the Jewish New Year, I patiently sat in the booth with my mother while they put the finishing touches on my new MAP. When they switched on the processor, I wasn't aware of any sounds at first, but I felt a sudden sensation in my head that sounded like the plucking of guitar strings for each syllable. The sound was awful, and I was shocked since it was not at all what I had anticipated. Initially, I was afraid and worried I had made a big mistake. I became very emotional. As I ventured out of the hospital, though, I noticed that everything made a sound. The scraping of the chair, the clanging of keys, shoes on the floor, the blaring of a P.A. system. Then outside came the honking, screeching brakes, sirens, and people yelling. It was truly overwhelming. Curiosity got the better of me and I asked my mother to identify each of those sounds as I pieced together a pattern. It was the beginning of therapy all over again.

After all these years, I went back for auditory rehabilitation at the Learning to Listen Foundation. Although the experience working with the therapists at LTLF was much different as an adult, the premise remained the same: to maximize my listening potential. We started off slowly with sounds, phrases, simple questions, and closed-set tasks before progressing to open-set tasks, conversation, and eventually talking on the telephone. This all took place over a period of 6–8 months.

It was a very difficult transition. At first, I thought the cochlear implant was a disaster. After some time, however, I realized the great potential and the wider range of sounds I was able to hear. It was a dream come true. I had more options than I had before. The day I picked up the phone, called my grandmother in Israel, and carried on a conversation with her without any assistance, we both cried.

Today, I can use the telephone, hear the doorbell, and listen to my son Jacob cry. The cochlear implant has enhanced the quality of my life. My experience also would lead my wife and my friend John to get implants of their own.

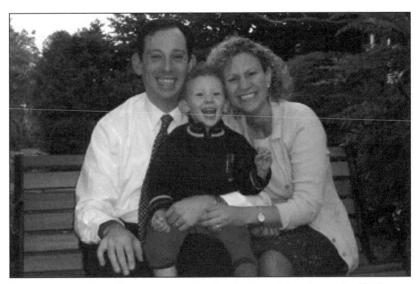

Because we rely heavily on our cochlear implants and hearing aids, Tania and I had concerns about interacting and communicating with our son Jacob, who was born deaf. We've found that our parenting is not affected.

Jacob's Promise

A big challenge came when Jacob was born. We had so many questions: How would we hear him at night? Would we be able to tell if he was sick? Would we hear what he was doing in the other room? Would we understand him? Would he understand us? All this meant further investigation into more technology. We probably have one of the most wired and wireless houses around. We now have three baby monitors: one equipped with a video camera perched over his crib, one with flashing lights to wake us up at night, and a third with a vibrator to carry around the house during the day. With the exception of the night monitor, these devices all complement our listening skills. We still rely heavily on our cochlear implants (and the hearing aids we use on our unimplanted ears).

Our concerns have been allayed, however. We have been able to interact and communicate with Jacob and understand his needs. Although we had our anxieties before he was born — not unlike any new parent — our hearing loss has not affected our parenting. In fact, we thankfully feel rather confident as parents.

Becoming a parent brought us a whole new set of responsibilities and worries. For one, would Jacob have normal hearing or would he be hearing impaired? We had our suspicions, which literally changed daily as we tried to determine whether he was responding to noise or not. At 3 weeks of age, we received the confirmation that Jacob was indeed profoundly deaf. Even though we were both devastated, we at least knew we could give Jacob the best any parent could offer because we had been through it ourselves. We recognized that 21st century technology was much better and that Jacob had many opportunities we hadn't had. This realization brought a new perspective. We redefined our relationships with various professionals, such as audiologists and teachers, and sought out our own support networks. We learned about the process.

Jacob was immediately fitted with hearing aids and we set out to work to communicate with him by pointing out as many sounds as possible despite his young age. We knew right away that the aids were giving him only limited information and that a cochlear implant would provide a stronger foundation for his listening and speaking skills. We also knew that it would make life much easier for him. Therefore, we had him evaluated and he indeed qualified for an implant. At 8 months of age, Jacob had his surgery, with activation a month later. It was almost as though a light bulb had been switched on. All of a sudden, it was the sounds that couldn't keep up with Jacob. He thrived in a world of clear and plentiful sounds. Any musical toy he had previously ignored promptly became his favorite. His body would swing to the beat as a huge grin crossed his face. Every morning and every afternoon after his nap, we would put the cochlear implant on him and his face would break into a smile. He just couldn't get enough sound, speech, or music. He has accomplished in the short postactivation period what it took years for me to do.

Jacob takes after his mother with a very social, bubbly personality. He loves to be around people and is very active and friendly. He attends several programs each week and enjoys playing with other children. He is interactive and likes to communicate and listen to us as we sing, talk, and read books with him.

Jacob, Tania, and I are currently enrolled in Auditory-Verbal therapy at the Learning to Listen Foundation. This is a second generation experience for us. We know first hand that A-V therapy is a commitment, but we also realize it will open as many doors for Jacob as possible. Just as my parents did with me, Tania and I feel strongly that Jacob is no different than anyone else, and we will always expect the best for him and from him.

Our journey with Jacob is just beginning, but the road will be familiar. We have made the following promises and commitments to our son:

- ❦ We promise to help you become as independent and confident as possible so you can advocate for yourself.
- ❦ We will provide the tools for you to do so.
- ❦ We will give you every chance to develop your listening potential, and your language and communication skills.
- ❦ We will empower you to become an active participant in taking care of yourself and your needs.
- ❦ We will never take a back seat. We will open many doors and offer you many paths from which to choose.
- ❦ We will enrich your life with our culture, heritage, and knowledge.
- ❦ We will be proud of your successes and guide you in learning from your failures.
- ❦ We will make learning fun, stimulating, and purposeful.
- ❦ We will provide you all our encouragement, love, and support.

CHAPTER 2

Karen

Karen MacIver-Lux

On May 15, 1971, my very quick arrival into this world was announced with the traditional "It's a girl!" My mother was elated, of course, and responded, "Oh boy!" The doctor quickly corrected her with an exuberant-sounding "Oh girl!" My mother saw me very briefly, clouded through eyes of happiness and exhaustion, and although the doctor sounded bright and cheerful, it was to keep my mother oblivious to the fact that something had gone terribly wrong.

Although her pregnancy had been uneventful, in the final weeks of gestation my mother had developed a mild case of toxemia. Despite this, she carried me to full term and went into labor while watching my brothers at their swimming lessons at the local community center. She managed to drive herself and my brothers to the hospital, where I was delivered 20 minutes later. Unaware that she had delivered the placenta first, her long-awaited newborn daughter arrived. Already blessed with two sons, she was simply elated that I was a girl and was not overly concerned when the delivery team rushed me away.

Unbeknownst to my mother, I was fighting for my life in the neonatal intensive care unit. Upon delivery, I had aspirated the amniotic fluid and was not breathing. The doctors were able to revive me, but were uncertain whether I was going to make it through the night. I was placed in an isolette and treated for pneumonia. Several rooms away, my mother was settling in for the night when she was interrupted by the news that her baby would probably not survive. All joy vanished. Deep fear and depression set in.

I made it through the first night and was appropriately nicknamed "the miracle baby." The doctors reminded my mother that each night I lived, my chances of long-term survival grew stronger. Every morning, my mother would eagerly await the news that I had made it through the night. After eight days in the neonatal intensive care unit, the doctors determined that I would fully recover. For the first time, my parents felt their dreams had been fulfilled, that the little girl they had always wanted was a reality.

Under the care of my mother and the hospital, I continued to make progress. Eventually, I was allowed to go home. Before discharge, however, the doctors informed my mother that they were uncertain as to just how the trauma I suffered would affect me. There were possibilities of mental retardation or problems with eyesight, but hearing loss was never mentioned.

A Hidden Hearing Loss

Despite all those troubles as a newborn, I thrived as an infant. I'm told I was a bundle of joy, and the object of my older brothers' adoration. David was 8 years old and was convinced he was his baby sister's "second daddy." Steven, meanwhile, doted on me as well as any 5-year-old boy could manage.

With the doctors' warnings swirling in her mind, my mother watched vigilantly for any sign of blindness and mental retardation. Although it was too early to tell about my mental capacities, she did note that my eyes were bright and always wide open — almost cartoon-like, she said — and I was quick to respond to any movement. I met all developmental milestones and seemed to be a normal and healthy baby girl.

> My mother noted I was quick to respond to any movement. I met all development milestones and seemed to be a normal and healthy girl.

Both my brothers were slow in learning to speak, but they eventually caught up to their peers by the time they were 4. Consequently, my parents weren't concerned when I hadn't said any words by 17 months of age. At 18 months, however, my mother said she noticed that when I was at the piano, I preferred playing the bass keys. She said that if I played a key at the upper end of the piano, I would pound the keys in frustration. When my mother came to stop me, I would babble angrily to her as if to say, "It's broken!" At that point, my mother wondered about my hearing and made an appointment to see our family doctor.

During the examination, the doctor propped me up on the table and conducted the clap test. I immediately rewarded him with consistent head turns in response to the clapping, and he promptly informed my mother that nothing was wrong with my hearing. Relieved, she took me home.

Over time, however, my mother continued to worry. Whenever she asked me to retrieve a particular toy or to put on a piece of clothing, I would always bring her the wrong items. I appeared to be bright, and in all other aspects of my development I seemed to be on schedule. She said I was quick to learn and very eager to please; thus, I would burst into tears every time she shook her head to indicate that I had brought the wrong item. Whenever I attempted to talk, it sounded like gibberish with only long vowel sounds. Whenever anyone asked me a question, I would reply with a poorly approximated version of the same question. Concerns about my hearing continued to resurface and my mother would dutifully take me back to the doctor. Again and again, the doctor tried to allay her fears by assuring her there was nothing wrong.

Eager to help with my delayed speech and language skills, my mother became convinced that the solution was to expose me to other children my age. She felt that by modeling their speech I would learn to talk clearly, so by the time I was 3, I was enrolled in every available toddler program in our

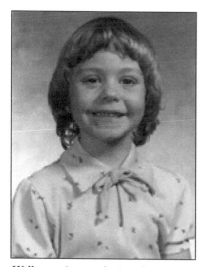

Well-meaning professionals said I would never learn to speak or be educated at a level higher than third grade, and that I might be able to get a job as a laborer. This was unacceptable to my mother.

community, including figure skating, baton twirling, and nursery school.

I have vague memories of being a 3-year-old. It seemed that I was always being touched, tugged, or rushed to go different places. I craved my family's familiar faces and my familiar routines. When I was exposed to new situations, I felt as though I was in a fast-motion black-and-white movie. The world seemed colorless. People would suddenly appear and disappear, suddenly look puzzled or annoyed, and then they would tug me here or there. I remember feeling helpless and frustrated because I could never seem to please anyone. Most of the time, I looked miserable. The only things that made me smile or laugh were the silly antics of my brothers, and the sight of Sausee, our standard smooth-haired Dachshund. My favorite place was in the arms of my mother or father, where their smiles and kisses offered comfort and acceptance. With my family's love and the routine of the toddler programs, I came to understand what was expected of me in a world full of unknowns.

My mother's fears about my hearing resurfaced continually. One month before my fourth birthday, she couldn't stand her nagging doubts any longer. Encouraged by her friend, a nurse who also suspected I might be deaf, my mother took me to the family doctor again and demanded to see both an ear, nose and throat (ENT) specialist and an audiologist. The doctor finally relented and referred us to the ENT, who performed the clap test and proclaimed my hearing to be "just fine." My mother insisted, however, that an audiologist give me a hearing test — just to be sure. He tested my hearing twice that day and it was then that her fears about my hearing were confirmed. She was told that I had a moderate-to-profound sensorineural hearing loss.

The audiologist suggested they send me to the Hospital for Sick Children in Toronto to get a prescription for hearing aids. There, a team of well-meaning professionals informed my mother that even with hearing aids my future was bleak. I would never learn to speak, they said. I would have to be sent away to a residential school for the deaf to learn sign language. I would never be educated at a level higher than third grade. When I was older, I might be able to earn a living as a laborer in a factory. Needless to say, this was all unacceptable to my mother. She ignored their recommendations and insisted that I be given a prescription for hearing aids right away and that I be fitted immediately. She even promised that she would return when I was speaking just to show those doctors what was possible.

Although she put on a brave face at the hospital, my mother was devastated. My father, on the other hand, had already experienced deafness while growing up (having a babysitter who was deaf). He was concerned, but he was relieved to discover that hearing loss, not mental retardation, was the reason for my obvious communication difficulties. He also felt my mother was more than capable of helping me learn to talk. However, despite my father's encouragement, my mother fell into the initial stages of grieving. Then one night, I became very ill and was taken to the hospital. Although my illness was not life-threatening, the experience reminded my mother that there are worse things in life than a diagnosis of deafness. As soon as I returned home in good health, she set to work on finding a therapist who would be willing to teach me to talk.

A Colorful World of Sound

My parents insisted that I be fitted with the latest in hearing aid technology. Behind-the-ear (BTE) hearing aids had just become available to the public in the 1970s. I distinctly remember the day I was fitted. I recall the pain as the audiologist tugged at my ears and inserted the earmolds. I remember bursting into tears as I saw the firm look in my mother's eyes which I understood to mean that these things in my ears were there to stay. I remember waving goodbye to the audiologist and leaving the office, which seemed to glow in golden yellow.

The first time I recall hearing sound was the crinkling of the plastic rain hat that my mother placed over my head. She was worried that the raindrops would get on my hearing aids, so she placed her hands over the hat that covered my ears. I have no recollection of the ride home on the subway train, but my mother certainly does. As soon as the train began moving, she said I began to scream and cry hysterically. My mother tried to calm me down without success. She said it wasn't until we got off the subway train that my crying and screaming subsided. She realized that it was the first time I had heard the sound of a train. I had been terrified.

My mother said that by the time I got to the car I was a different girl. Her previously miserable little daughter had slowly and gently turned into a girl full of laughter. She was amazed at the transformation. I would coo, then laugh, obviously delighted with the sound of my own voice. I remember being amused by the "new" sounds I could make and the noise of the car as it struggled to start. The car, it seemed, had begun to glow in cornflower blue.

On the evening of my first "hearing day," I had my first baton rehearsal and heard music clearly for the first time. As the opening bars of "Raindrops Keep Falling on My Head" played, I stood still in complete awe as my classmates twirled their batons. I suddenly understood why everyone was moving around in perfect synchrony. The music stirred my emotions, and as I celebrated my newest discovery, the mothers in the audience wept. From that moment, the black-and-white movie of life became a Technicolor® motion picture. Life seemed to become richer and brighter. The door to my world of sound had opened and I was ready to embark on a new journey.

Learning to Listen and Talk at an Early Age

My mother joined a parent support group in Toronto known as VOICE for Hearing Impaired Children (VOICE), whose vision was that children with hearing loss could learn to listen and talk. Shortly after joining, she attended a conference where Daniel Ling was a principal speaker. Dr. Ling was a prominent leader in the development of spoken communication for children who were deaf or hard of hearing. Among the topics he discussed at the conference was the importance of helping children who are deaf to develop listening skills using advanced hearing technology. He emphasized the importance of listening first — not lipreading — because many sounds look the same on the lips.

My mother was inspired. She was determined that this was the approach that would help me learn to talk. She found a speech-language pathologist at a local hospital who would provide therapy for me. This therapist was a recent university graduate who, along with my mother, was willing to learn about the Ling Method. Since my attention span seemed exceptional, my mother was able to talk the therapist into giving me a 2-hour therapy session twice a week. She spent the first hour-and-a-half in direct therapy with us, and the remaining half-hour providing guidance for my mother.

I loved therapy sessions with my therapist. She had a knack for making listening and talking fun. My favorite lessons were about prepositions. When I was learning about *on*, both of us would sit on the therapy table and play games. When I was learning about *under*, we had a tea party under the table. We worked under the table for an entire week, in fact. Through my therapist, my mother learned how to make language-learning natural.

At home, every action or event was narrated. My mother talked and talked for me — I don't ever remember her being quiet. She made sure I was by her side at all times, so not a moment of language learning was missed. (She made sure I was close to her so I could hear her well.) In retrospect, I don't know how she did it. When the house chores were talked about and done, it was time for *sit-down* therapy. I remember sitting on a plastic covered chair for an hour, sometimes two, working hard on speech sounds that were difficult for me to hear and say such as *ch*, *r*, and *s*. When I would finish, my backside would seem molded permanently into the chair, and my mother and I would laugh at the sound it would make as I stood up.

She read many children's books with me and made "experience" books with crayons, craft items, and glue. On a chalkboard in the kitchen, she would draw pictures and write out key vocabulary words and letters of the alphabet. Although I remember the experiences and materials, I don't remember ever thinking of it as work. My mother tells me that I could sit for hours. The patience and perseverance I showed in attempting to correctly produce those harder-to-hear speech sounds amazed her. When she was frustrated because I couldn't get a sound no matter how often I tried, I would comfort her with a pat on her back, saying, "It's OK, Mommy."

At home, every action or event was narrated. My mother talked and talked for me – I don't ever remember her being quiet.

Determined that I would learn not only to speak but also to read, every object in the house was labeled. I learned quickly that if I wanted to do something or use something, I would have to first use my words to the best of my ability. My mother always raised the bar by challenging me to do better.

Eventually, the gibberish turned into clear words, phrases, and sentences that clearly communicated my observations, wants, and needs. Although my pronunciation was far from perfect, strangers normally could understand me. My parents, of course, were elated by my progress.

My family has fond memories of miscommunications that often resulted from my inability either to hear or speak clearly. These often had my family members doubling over with laughter while I stood there with my hands up in the air. There is one situation I remember vividly, however. When I was 7, I was introduced to Shirley Temples and delighted at eating the cherry and orange that accompanied the drink. At that age, I could order for myself at restaurants and usually had no difficulty in getting my point across until it was time to order the Shirley Temple. The waiters and waitresses usually asked me to repeat my request several times and, once they figured out what it was I wanted to drink, they typically walked off with a chuckle. My brothers would then snicker and my mother would slap them and smile sweetly at me. This became a common occurrence every time we went to a restaurant. Two years later, we were eating in a restaurant owned by a family friend. After I ordered the drink, our friend shook his head at my mother and said, "I can't take this anymore!" He took my chin in his hand and said slowly, "Karen, it's not cherry pimple, it's Shirley Temple!" I turned to my mother in anger and asked her why she would let me make such a mistake for so long. "But Karen," she responded. "I thought it was so cute!"

To this day, I continue to make mistakes, but instead of cringing in embarrassment, I now let go and have a good laugh about them. I've found that repeating what I heard often makes my communication partner laugh. Not only does this lighten up a potentially tense situation, it also helps my partner understand that although I listen well with my hearing aids, I still make mistakes.

Choosing a Mainstream Education

After about a year of therapy, my parents began to think seriously about my educational future. They were firm in their decision not to send me away to a residential school for the deaf; they wanted me in the neighborhood school with my friends who were good speech and language models. The principal of the school, however, had other ideas on how I should obtain my education. The school for the deaf, he asserted, was the right place for me.

In the early 1970s, the world experienced a boom in hearing aid and assistive listening device technology. One example was the Phonic Ear® body-worn FM system, which was particularly beneficial in the classroom setting. This device consisted of a microphone/transmitter worn by the teacher and a receiver worn by the child on his or her chest. The FM system was designed to help the child clearly hear the primary speech signal (i.e., the teacher's voice) while eliminating or reducing the background environmental or speech noise.

My mother was interested in obtaining an FM system for me, but she was strongly advised against it by an experienced parent from VOICE who reasoned that the device was a "crutch." At that time, the efficacy of the Phonic Ear system had not been proved, so my mother decided to defer its purchase until more definitive data were available.

On a return flight from a business trip with my father, my mother happened to notice that the man in the seat beside her had brochures about the Phonic Ear system. She introduced herself and told the man about me, only to discover that he was a Phonic Ear representative. She expressed her concerns that I might use the system as a crutch, to which he replied, "Mrs. MacIver, don't you think your daughter needs all the crutches she can get?" He told my mother that the Toronto District School Board had initiated a study to prove the efficacy of the FM system and its use in the classroom. The study would involve 50 children with hearing loss who would be mainstreamed into regular classrooms with an FM system and an itinerant teacher of the deaf to provide support services three times a week. For the first time, their hopes and dreams that I receive my education in a typical classroom were on the verge of becoming a reality.

Report cards from kindergarten to fourth grade document not only my progress in academics but also my language development. In kindergarten, I was able to say the names of many of my classmates clearly, and I enjoyed singing games with other children. My ability to concentrate improved when my hearing aids were turned on. I put a lot of effort into listening during all lessons and discussions. My oral language became more coherent, and new vocabulary and sentence structures developed satisfactorily. In first grade, my oral language improved steadily. I liked to express my ideas, but I needed to listen more carefully to questions before answering them. I loved to sing songs and could tone-match quite well. By third grade, I could read at my grade level, but my skills in mathematics were poor: I couldn't figure out whether to add or subtract in word problems.

> Although my class-mates accepted me, I didn't make close friends easily. Perhaps it was because I was linguistically and socially naive.

In fourth grade, I had a teacher from Scotland. His accent was very difficult for me to understand, and my academics and listening skills suffered as a result. Regarding my language, he commented: "This whole area is, of course, greatly affected by Karen's hearing loss. Creative writing is still at a primary level, with difficulties in grammar usage further complicated by omissions." After seeing this report card, my parents decided to take me out of the class and enroll me in the Toronto Learning Center in order to get me up to grade level. That was a very positive experience. The classes were small and there were several teachers for each classroom, which were carpeted and had walls covered in fabric so it was easy for me to hear.

Although my classmates accepted me at the various schools I attended, I didn't make close friends easily. Perhaps it was because I was linguistically and socially naive. Or perhaps it was because I spent much of the school day away from the classroom attending extra speech lessons and sessions with a teacher of the deaf. I do remember that I never felt "different" from other children. In retrospect, I think Hollywood played a significant role in helping my classmates accept me with my hearing aids and FM system. In the 1970s, there was a popular television show called "The Six Million Dollar Man" whose main character had bionic parts that made him superhuman. To help inquiring peers understand what my hearing aid was, my mother explained that I had a "bionic ear." I was thrilled with my "bionic ear" and felt proud to wear it. And, according to my mother, my classmates were equally in awe.

In 1981, my father accepted a senior position with a company based in Alberta. Therefore, in the summer between fourth and fifth grades, my family moved to Calgary. My parents were excited at the chance to begin a new life out west. I was excited about the chance to begin life on prairie soil. A voracious reader, I loved my *Little House on the Prairie* books and was eager to experience the land of the pioneers. My only disappointment was that we were not moving out west in a covered wagon.

My parents' excitement was not to last long. Officials at the local public school were reluctant to accept me as a student and suggested that I instead attend a school for the deaf. After being denied entrance on the first day of school, my mother and I walked home in tears. Later that afternoon, the principal of the school received a phone call from my father. That call was enough to change the principal's mind and the next day I began school with my personal FM system.

> Officials at the local public school were reluctant to accept me. After being denied entrance on the first day, my mother and I walked home in tears.

Despite these initial difficulties, my year in Calgary turned out to be the best year of my childhood. I was blessed with an outstanding teacher who took pride in the fact that he had me in his classroom. He enjoyed wearing the FM transmitter, and he made sure that my classmates understood why I wore hearing aids and used the FM system. He took special interest in helping me with subjects in which I had traditionally struggled. I blossomed under his tutelage.

I also became fast friends with three girls with hearts of gold. Tania was an established model with one of Canada's foremost modeling agencies; Meagan was the sophisticated and mature one; and Kim was a lover of books and sports just like me. We were the *preteen sensations,* doing everything together. With the help of our parents, we held fashion shows in our homes, had bake sales to fund our shopping trips, and often shopped without supervision in the area malls. For our birthdays, we went to restaurants on our own while our nervous parents waited in their cars in the parking lot. Our friendships helped me develop the confidence, strength, and courage to deal with what would become some of the most difficult years of my life.

After a year in Calgary, my father decided it was time to move back to Toronto — a traumatic move for me. I was homesick for the mountains and the best friends I had left behind in Calgary. I couldn't hear very well on the phone, so I couldn't keep in touch with them. I remember them calling me and trying to comfort me, but I was unable to understand their words. Every night, it seemed, I would dream of meeting them in an open field where we would try to speak, but for some reason our voices wouldn't reach one another. I would wake up in tears and my mother would rock me as I cried. For the first time in my life, I truly felt hurt by what I considered the limitations of hearing loss.

Life went on and I was determined to make new friends. My mother and I decided it would be good to attend a summer camp close to our cottage in Muskoka, Ontario. At the camp, there was a girl in my cabin who would be in my sixth-grade class in the fall. We quickly became close friends and eagerly planned the fun times we would have together in school.

I began sixth grade without my FM system since it was being reconditioned at the manufacturer. The week I waited for it to arrive back was a long one. All seemed well, however, as I was able to make friends with the "popular" group of kids at school, and the teachers were supportive and welcomed my inclusion in their classes. However, when I appeared the second week of school with my newly repaired FM system, right away I felt eyes upon me, and my new "friends" quickly turned their backs on me. I was confused and hurt and couldn't understand the change in their attitudes. I wasn't kept in the dark for long as notes started to appear in my desk and pencil bag: *Bag your face! Go away! Deaf and Dumb!* Cartoon pictures of me with wires coming out my ears were particularly hurtful. Worst of all, my friend from camp abandoned me.

The nightly crying episodes began again. I missed my friends in Calgary even more. I just couldn't understand why I was suddenly singled out as "unpopular." As each day went on, the popular crowd made life at school increasingly difficult. My self-esteem plummeted and my grades began to suffer. I became self-conscious of my hearing aids and FM system. At the same time, I was ashamed of myself for feeling self-conscious about the very things that were essential to my quality of life. The unpopular girls slowly began to reach out to me and I gravitated toward their friendship. Each of these girls had something about them that was discriminated against: weight, nationality, or socioeconomic status. With their help, I learned that it didn't matter what you were on the outside. It was what you were on the inside that counted much more. Some of these girls are still my friends today.

> When I appeared with my newly repaired FM system, my new 'friends' quickly turned their backs on me. I couldn't understand the change in attitude.

Despite having friends, the popular crowd continued to taunt me. For the first time in my life, I began to experience bitterness. The only thing I knew I could do to fight back was to irritate the student behind me by "accidentally" hitting him in the head with the shoulder straps of my FM system as I put it on. That, however, did little to stop the taunting. I cried my heart out to my mother, who could do nothing but listen and encourage me to face the next day. Luckily, I had ways to escape the tears because I was involved in many after-school activities: ballet, figure skating, swimming, and the church drama club. My parents felt these activities were essential in helping me maintain whatever confidence and positive self-image I had left — and they were right. Besides, I enjoyed the few hours of joy, peace, and acceptance that these hobbies offered.

My itinerant teacher, Anne, often came to school during lunch hours to offer respite from the nasty classmates. I would share my latest experiences and feelings, and she would share experiences she had growing up. It helped to hear what she went through and how she managed to cope with the teasing and taunting. She had great integrity and taught me to hold my head up and look the other way. She also reminded me daily of the power of kindness, humility, and respect for others no matter how bad the situation. For that, I will forever be grateful.

I had always struggled with vocabulary, reading comprehension, and math. Spelling and history were my best and, of course, favorite subjects. Anne introduced me to the thesaurus and the Canadian author Lucy Maud Montgomery. For my first reading assignment, she gave me Montgomery's *Emily of New Moon*, which remains one of my favorite books. I loved reading about Emily, a dreamer who never let adversity get her down. Anne tended to give me books that were about heroines who overcame serious obstacles in life, such as unpopularity or a disability. These heroines inspired me to become the best I could be.

Anne and my parents worked hard to instill in me a sense of responsibility to do my best in battling the difficulties I faced so that the next student with hearing loss who came along would have an easier time with his or her teachers or classmates. Anne and my parents were my support system and my cheerleaders. They strove to teach me to "kill my adversaries with kindness" and to "negotiate my way out of impossible situations."

> It was up to me to trick these classmates into thinking they no longer had the power to hurt or control me.

In seventh grade, my parents decided it was time I take charge of the troubling situation I faced at school since it was affecting my grades. One night, I showed them the latest batch of notes and pictures. My father told me it was important that I have a game plan to trick my opponents. My parents explained that my classmates had a game plan of their own, which was to make my life so miserable I would leave the school and never return. It was up to me to trick these classmates into thinking they no longer had the power to hurt or control me.

I quickly got to work pasting all the notes and pictures on a board, and my mother had it professionally framed by a family friend. I planned to take the framed picture to school and wait until lunch to launch my counterattack. What made this plan so brilliant was the fact that the class ate in the classroom with the teacher. One day, I retrieved my picture and stood up on my chair where everyone could not help but notice me. I held up the picture and proceeded with my carefully planned speech.

"I just wanted to thank everyone in the class for helping me create this lovely picture," I said. "Some of you love me so much that you actually spent the time and energy during class to write these love notes and draw terrific pictures of me. I love these notes and pictures so much that I decided to put them together and have them framed. I will hang this up on my bedroom wall so that every morning I can wake up and see this picture, and be reminded of how lucky I am that I have such loving classmates. Thanks, guys!"

I jumped off my chair and made a move to return the frame to my locker when the teacher called me to her desk. She asked if she could have a look at the picture and I proudly presented it to her. After carefully reviewing each note and picture, she handed the frame back to me. I saw a look of respect in her eyes, and she simply smiled. After that day, I never got another note.

Learning the Language of Possibilities

By the time I was 11, my mother decided I should change therapists. In six years, I had had three speech-language pathologists. My mother kept in touch with Dr. Ling from time to time so he could check on my progress and for his suggestions on goals for listening, speech, language, and my academics in general. Through Dr. Ling and VOICE, my mother learned about a young therapist named Warren Estabrooks. After hearing so many parents sing songs of praise about him and his therapeutic approach, my mother was determined that I should see him. When she called to make an appointment, however, she was informed that I was too old to receive Auditory-Verbal therapy at North York General Hospital, where Warren worked. My mother persisted and I was finally accepted into the A-V program on the condition I could prove to Warren that I, not my mother, wanted to have this therapy. He was the first professional to expect me to take

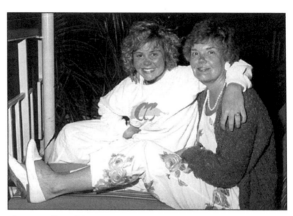

Originally told I was too old for Auditory-Verbal therapy, my mother persisted until I was accepted, on the condition I could prove I wanted the therapy.

charge of my listening and speaking skills. It was up to me, not my parents, to *want* to make positive changes in my life. I felt empowered for the first time.

My primary therapist was Cathy, but Warren worked with me from time to time. First, we worked on improving my listening skills. I was having trouble with solving oral (not written) math problems since I couldn't retain the critical information in the problem long enough to know whether to add, subtract, multiply, or divide to get the solution. Warren noticed right away that I needed better hearing aids. He recommended a model from a hearing aid company whose brand I continue to wear today. What a difference! I remember sitting in my bedroom and hearing a constant whishing noise that I had never heard before. I remember telling my mother excitedly that I could hear the air, only to have her laugh and tell me that it was the highway traffic two blocks away.

Cathy introduced me to a different form of articulation therapy. She had me record myself talking and encouraged me to listen to my speech as it played through the tape player. I was so motivated to speak well during therapy sessions that she struggled to find things on which to work. I remember Cathy looking at my mother and saying, "Sheila, she's doing so well. She doesn't need the therapy!" My mother would respond, "But, she sounds horrible at home. She doesn't talk like this at all!" I remember feeling rather smug and proud of myself. Then Cathy and my mother would engage me in a conversation about figure skating or my classmates and the true caliber of my speech would come through.

At that time, I was shy around older and handsome men. At times, I would give Warren my "cool" attitude, which would often come off sounding like a teenager with a "bad" attitude. I truly admired and respected my therapists at NYGH for the respect they showed me. Warren often spoke to me first and would always find some way to challenge me to do better, not only with my listening skills but also with my self-worth. I had dreams of becoming an audiologist, which most people scoffed at. How could a girl who is deaf become an audiologist?

Near the end of my block of therapy, Warren recommended to my mother that she begin helping me to listen on the telephone. I was very reluctant to try using the phone, having struggled to do so in the past. Warren was adamant that I give it another try, and he was quite persistent and stubborn about this issue. My mother quickly emulated his stubbornness. I cried, pleaded, and threatened as best I could, but to no avail. She arranged to have a new phone line installed in our house, with my monthly baby bonus check from the Canadian government used to pay the bill.

My telephone training began with a call from my mother. Three months later, I was confident enough to try calling my best friend. It wasn't long before we were talking for hours.

Satisfied that I had reached my listening and spoken communication potential, I graduated from the Auditory-Verbal therapy program at NYGH. Initially, my mother and I were nervous to be cut loose from the ship that had given us so much support. But we understood that it was time to move on and make room for other young children trying to learn to listen and talk.

Taking Advantage of a Private Education

When it was time to begin secondary school, my parents decided to send me to the Toronto District Christian High School (TDCH), a private school in Woodbridge. I was upset and told my parents very firmly that I would attend no such school. I wanted to go to the local public high school with the few friends I had. My parents explained my options: If I chose to go to the local school, my current classmates would be there, but if the going got tough, I would not be allowed to switch schools. But if I tried TDCH first and found I didn't like it, then I would be allowed to transfer to the local school. I thought seriously about my decision and even spoke to my brother Steven, who had just graduated from the public high school. He said I should take advantage of a private education where my marks would count more for university. I would have good teachers, he said, and students would more likely be free from the alcohol and drug problems that plagued the public school system. It was his one final comment, however, that ultimately helped me decide. He told me he would be disappointed if I chose to pass on the chance of a private education. I adored my brother and didn't want to disappoint him! I knew he wanted the best for me.

Looking back, I have no regrets. I admit my parents and my brother were right. I had an easier time making friends in high school and I steered clear of those who I perceived were part of the "popular" crowd. Although those kids did nothing to exclude me, I chose to exclude myself from that circle. I realize now I might have missed opportunities to establish some lasting friendships, but I didn't want to risk being hurt again. At the time, I felt it best to be part of a small group.

One of the consequences of attending a private school was that services from the public school board would discontinue. By attending TDCH, I lost the weekly support provided by an itinerant teacher of the deaf. Initially, my grades suffered because I missed deadlines for assignments and didn't know how to study for tests on my own. I had become dependent on my itinerant teacher since she made sure that I met all project deadlines and that I was properly prepared to pass tests. Going to school on my own proved to be a real awakening.

My mother enlisted the support of my other older brother, David, who was attending the University of Toronto. David sat me down and explained the responsibility involved in taking my own notes during class and the importance of keeping track of assignments, deadlines, and test dates. At the time, David was dating a nursing student, Julie, who would become his wife. I admired her and learned by example from her how to take notes and organize myself.

My mother decided to volunteer as assistant librarian at TDCH. She already was busy as president of her own music management and publishing company, and everyone at school knew that my mother and I went to bars, recording studios, and concerts to listen to rock groups and musicians seeking representation. Because she was considered "cool," I didn't mind her presence in the library.

Volunteering at school turned out to be a wise decision for my mother. It gave her immediate access to my teachers, and they aproached her in private to discuss their concerns about my "unrealistic and high expectations for taking advanced level courses that would gain entrance to University." Since my grades were not impressive in my first term in high school, my mother had to work hard to convince them I wasn't in over my head. The teachers agreed to allow me to continue taking advanced level courses as long as my grades improved. With my family's support, I finally learned to take responsibility for my own education, and my grades slowly improved. I worked hard to achieve my dream of attending university.

Following the Music

Our home was always filled with music. My mother descended from a long line of musicians and artists, and she became a music teacher. She believed that music and singing would help me attain clear, natural-sounding speech, so she always sang and played the piano, hoping that I would follow her lead. As a lover of music myself, it was never difficult to lure me to the beauty of music. An early favorite was slow classical music, to which I loved to hum along. In dance classes, I enjoyed both classical music and popular musicians such as the Bee Gees and Rod Stewart. On the long road trips we would take, I grew to adore Barbara Streisand and Bette Midler, as well as groups such as Bread and ABBA. Since my brothers enjoyed heavy metal groups such as Kiss and Van Halen, I was also exposed to that musical genre.

Today, I find it easier to hear and appreciate slower-paced music. It takes me longer to learn to appreciate and recognize the melody of songs that are fast and more complex. Also, it is impossible for me to hear the lyrics in many songs, so I depend on reading them. Once I have read the lyrics, the songs are easier to follow and sing along to.

For me, music evokes bright flashes of brilliant colors that appear and disappear in rhythm and pattern. It stirs my emotions and has the power to lift me amazingly. It gives me the courage to continue on when I get discouraged and helps me celebrate my successes.

For as long as I can remember, I took piano lessons. Although I loved listening to music and creating my own tunes, I wasn't a very good student. Music teachers always seemed to think in mathematical terms, and I could never understand those whole, half, and quarter pies they used to draw on paper. What did pies have to do with music, anyway? Before I learned to play a new song, they would play the song themselves. And, by memory, I would play the notes just as they did. However, I was terrible at reading music.

It wasn't until I was in fifth grade that my mother realized the teachers were trying — unsuccessfully — to teach me about apple and cherry pies. She took me out of those classes and taught me through listening about quarter, half, and whole notes. I realized then that they represented the pattern and timing of music. This made sense to me. My piano lessons went much better after that.

I joined a hand bell choir and learned to listen for my cues. I was able to handle five hand bells and could switch them quickly as needed.

I also joined a hand bell choir. I learned to listen to the other hand bells as they were played and to listen for my cues to play. I was able to handle five hand bells and could switch them quickly as the music progressed. I loved participating in what became an award-winning choir.

I learned to play the trumpet, too, and played in the school bands throughout junior and senior high school. Playing the trumpet helped strengthen my breathing skills and, in turn, helped improve the quality of my voice.

Throughout high school, I sang in the choir. Music teachers were amazed that I could sing on key. My voice was always a bit weak, but it improved when I had lessons from an opera singer who was a good family friend. We worked on improving my breathing skills and spent many hours doubled up in laughter after she would have me sing while I hung upside down from the back of the church pews.

In high school, I spent considerable time studying and completing my homework in recording studios. My mother had a great interest in helping young musicians. She would teach them and arrange lessons with more established musicians. I found it fascinating to learn how music was recorded, instrument by instrument, track by track, until a song was completed. I learned to appreciate the musical gifts that each instrument offered, and how timing was everything in ensuring that the music flowed together.

By spending some of my formative years in the music industry, I was able to heal some of the emotional wounds I had received in grade school. I felt accepted by the musicians, and this went a long way in improving my self-esteem. I also learned that I wasn't alone in feeling rejected. I observed many rock bands recording demo tapes hoping to secure a contract with a major record company. Watching these musicians accept or reject constructive feedback from producers and engineers taught me a great deal about life. Rejection, I discovered, is a tool to help us look within ourselves to find and develop hidden talents we never thought we had. When the musicians finally landed recording contracts, they shared their success with me. I basked in the delight of their newfound celebrity, enjoyed the excitement of the Juno awards (the Canadian equivalent of the American Grammies), and the opportunity to meet popular Canadian musicians and bands.

Boys, Boys, Boys!

I was always infatuated with gorgeous boys who wanted to run a million miles away from me. But, most boys who came after me . . . well, I wanted to run a million miles from them! As a result, I remained dateless for the first few years of high school, which was fine with my overprotective father, though it wasn't fine with me.

Many times I sat with Steven and shared my heartache over the boys with whom I had fallen hopelessly in love. One day, I asked Steven if it was because of my hearing loss that guys I liked looked the other way. Steven answered honestly and said it was possible. However, he told me something that I never forgot. He said I should feel lucky to have hearing aids because they were great "jerk screeners." If the boys weren't men enough to look past the hearing aids to my heart, then they weren't worthy of my time, he said, before adding with a wink that it saved them from having to deal with a protective big brother.

My last year of high school, I began dating a boy a year older than me. We attended our high school proms together, and spent time at our cottages during the summer breaks. My parents were elated that I was dating him since he was a nice boy with healthy ambitions. Over time, however, we found that our ambitions and dreams differed, and our relationship ended.

The other dates I had were with older men, and I suspect that had a lot to do with their maturity and their ability to look beyond my hearing aids. They were kind, but I didn't see any sense in pursuing a relationship if I didn't think it was going anywhere. Each date and relationship prepared me well for finding the love of my life, but I first wanted to pursue the education and career of my dreams.

Building My Own Hopes and Dreams

My mother never did take me back to the Toronto hospital where I was born to prove wrong those professionals who said I would never talk or obtain higher than a third-grade education. We didn't have enough time for that.

She prepared me for independence in subtle ways. The first test came when it was time to get my driver's license. My mother insisted that I make the phone call to the driving school myself. I refused to do it and she refused to do it for me. She argued that if I was old enough to drive, then I was old enough to register myself for courses. I begged, pleaded, and used every excuse in the book. My mother held her ground. After a year of waiting and building the courage, I finally made the phone call to Young Drivers of Canada. That call took no more than five minutes. The secretary was very pleasant and easy to understand. I was angry with myself for waiting so long. I felt proud that I had done it on my own. I am extremely grateful for the independence I enjoy from using the telephone.

I obtained my first job when I was 15, working in a small clothing store during my summer break. Over the next few years, I contributed to my savings by working at summer and weekend jobs. I learned the importance of a work ethic and accepting constructive criticism. In my final two years of high school, I worked at a large home builder's store where I held positions of responsibility in the administrative department and was trusted to handle sensitive financial documents. I learned how to manage conflicts at the employee and administrative level. Most important, I learned to listen and interact well with customers so their needs could be met.

As a high school senior, I was accepted into the Communication Disorders Program at a satellite campus of Purdue University in Fort Wayne, Indiana (IPFW). To prepare for my studies in communication disorders, I volunteered at my audiologist's office several evenings a week, filing audiograms and preparing appointment sheets. My audiologist was extremely supportive of my career choice and we developed a plan to achieve my educational goals.

I began my studies at IPFW in the fall of 1990. I decided to live with family friends during the first semester in order to learn my way around and look for an affordable apartment.

> The program chair said she didn't know of any audiologists who were deaf and feared that I wouldn't be accepted to a graduate school program.

As I was leaving my first class in communication disorders, the professor notified me that the program chair wanted to see me. I proceeded to her office with trepidation, wearing a bright smile but preparing myself for the worst. The chair informed me that I had only been accepted into the program because I was an international student. She told me that majors were required to pass speech and hearing screening tests before they could continue studying in the program. My heart dropped since I knew I would fail both tests. I had to think fast on my feet. I asked her why such a policy existed and what her real concerns were. She was frank and said she didn't know of any audiologists who were deaf and was afraid that I wouldn't be accepted into a graduate school program because of my hearing loss. Rather than react with threats of discrimination lawsuits, however, I tried negotiating first. My offer? If I contacted several graduate schools and obtained letters guaranteeing acceptance as long as my grades met their academic criteria, would I be allowed to continue in the IPFW program? She thought for a moment and then nodded "yes." That "sounded fair enough to her."

I began setting up appointments. My first stop was with Dr. Goldstein, the chair of the Department of Audiology at Purdue's main campus. My mother came to support me at this interview. When I was called into the office, I was greeted by Dr. Goldstein and a young woman. I noticed right away that Dr. Goldstein wore hearing aids himself, which bolstered my confidence. As he introduced himself, the woman beside him began signing. I shook Dr. Goldstein's hand and thanked him for seeing me on such short notice. He looked quite surprised and inquired whether I knew sign language. I told him, "No, but I could learn." He dismissed the interpreter and asked for a copy of my transcript. After reviewing my grades for the first semester, he smiled and said, "You'll have no problem getting into the program if you maintain these grades." He wrote a letter of support and even suggested other programs I could visit for positive letters of recommendation.

I was allowed to continue my studies at IPFW, which had a strong clinical-based program. Consequently, I gained many hours of practical experience in audiology and speech-language pathology. I was asked to take on children with hearing loss for aural habilitation. I quickly discovered that not only did I love conducting hearing tests and hearing aid work, but I also loved working with children on aural habilitation. My professors recognized my interest and potential and allowed me to take on more clients. I had finally found my niche.

During my studies and clinical practica, I used my FM system faithfully. I kept my own notes and took the initiative to photocopy the notes of two classmates. Each night, I would rewrite my notes with added information from those of my classmates. This was an effective way for me to study and, as a result, I made the national dean's list for outstanding grades for several semesters. I also was a recipient of a *Who's Who in American Colleges and Universities* award.

In my independent studies in aural habilitation, I learned everything I could about Auditory-Verbal therapy. During my research, I came across Warren Estabrooks' name in articles associated with the Auditory-Verbal approach. I remember running to one of my professors to brag that he had been one of my teachers and was instrumental in helping me achieve the quality of life I now enjoyed.

At IPFW, I enjoyed wonderful friendships with several students who shared my major, and with two Canadian athletes attending IPFW on sport scholarships. The Canadians stuck together and formed a small patriotic group. I was the only girl in the group, and the two boys became my brothers-away-from-home. They watched over me and made sure that I took my head out of the books long enough to have some fun. I also watched over them and made sure they didn't get into trouble when they partied too hard. I constantly reminded them to pay more attention to their studies. When we were homesick for Swiss Chalet and Canadian beer, we drove home to Toronto for the long weekends. We made a great team.

Love of My Life

Love often comes when it's least expected . . . in the most unexpected way.

In my third year at IPFW, I moved in with Zorica and her husband Jim. Zorica's parents were from Croatia. Her mother had passed away a few years earlier, and her father was the only family she had in America. Zorica had an older sister, Dragenia, who was living in Berlin and who had just arrived in Chicago to meet her father. He called to say he was bringing Dragenia down to Fort Wayne.

Since Zorica was in the middle of exams and couldn't skip the class to meet her sister when she arrived, I had the pleasure of being the first person to meet Dragenia. I was excited for an opportunity to practice the few German phrases I had learned on my travels in Europe. The visit went well, and we concluded the afternoon with dinner at a local restaurant. Dragenia showed me pictures of her children, including one of her son Martin, and indicated through a combination of English and gesture that he had just broken up with his girlfriend. She inquired whether I would be interested in corresponding with him. Despite my polite decline, Dragenia promised that she would have her son write me a letter.

A month later, in October of 1992, I received a letter from Martin that included his picture. He wanted to know whether I would correspond with him, but I wasn't sure. I didn't see how I could have a pen pal relationship with someone who could barely write English. Zorica dragged me to a local Hallmark store and chose pretty stationary for my reply. She was determined that I write to her nephew, and I was more afraid of what would happen if I didn't. So I wrote Martin and included a very fuzzy picture of myself.

Two weeks later, I received a reply. Martin seemed very eager to learn more about me. He wanted to have my telephone number so he could call. Panic began to set in. I was sure that this was not going to work. Me, on the phone, with a guy who could barely speak a word of English? I had trouble enough with people with slight accents, and I couldn't see myself being friends with someone who couldn't speak my own language. I ignored his request for my telephone number and hoped that with a new and clearer picture of me he would forget about making that call.

I hadn't told Martin that I was hearing impaired. I wondered what he might think – if he would feel cheated or lied to. I kept putting it off.

I went home for Christmas break and spent the holiday with my family at our cottage. While I was out skiing with my brother Steven, Martin telephoned the cottage and ended up talking to my sister-in-law and my mother. Excited that a man from Germany was calling for me, my mother promised that I would call him back on Christmas day. I came home from my skiing trip to find my mother and sister-in-law jumping excitedly. My heart dropped when my mother told me she had promised Martin that I would call him back. I was furious! I began my excuses and pleadings, but, as usual, they fell on "deaf" ears. At 3 the next morning, my mother stood over my bed with the phone in her hand and a very defiant look in her eyes. I shooed her out of the room and dialed Martin's telephone number. Somehow, I didn't seem to have too much difficulty understanding him. We spoke in broken English for 30 minutes and I promised that I would call him when I returned to Fort Wayne.

In the new year, we began weekly telephone calls. There was something about Martin that held my interest. The whole situation seemed impossible, but whenever I spoke to him it seemed so right and natural. Martin worked hard to learn English over the telephone and during his free time. He proved to be a quick learner. The oddest thing was that other people had difficulty understanding him, but I didn't. I began to think that God was guiding me toward him.

As our relationship developed, I began to feel guilty. I hadn't told Martin that I was hearing impaired. I wondered what he might think — if he would feel cheated or lied to. I kept putting it off since I was afraid he would lose interest in me once he found out. I agonized over whether I should tell him then or later. Zorica's husband Jim finally stepped in and put a stop to my nonsense. His words echoed my brother's: If Martin was not man enough to accept your hearing loss, then he was not worth your time. He added that it was important that I be positive and upbeat. My attitude would be important in his willingness to accept me as I was.

I wrote Martin a long letter explaining my hearing loss, my hearing aids, and the career I had chosen. Martin called me as soon as he received the letter and told me he loved me just the way I was and that it was just fine with him. He did wonder how I could hear and speak so well on the phone. He thought it both incredible and amazing. His positive response went a long way in reassuring me about my feelings for him.

In July, I flew to Germany to meet Martin for the first time. That October, Martin visited me in Indiana and we became engaged. The following May, he emigrated to Canada, just in time to watch me graduate from IPFW with a bachelor of science degree.

Finding My Dreams

In the fall, I moved on to the University of Akron to begin my graduate studies, while Martin stayed in Toronto to earn his diploma in business administration at Humber College. He also took courses at York University to improve his spoken and written English. Each weekend, he would drive five hours to Akron to visit me. We supported each other in our studies and in our plans for the future.

The University of Akron offered an outstanding graduate program in audiology. The faculty included some of the nation's most respected audiologists, and the facilities were quite modern, with up-to-date testing equipment. Most important, I was there to learn from Carol Flexer, whose work I deeply respect. Dr. Flexer had just been elected president of the American Academy of Audiology and had gained international recognition for her work in educational and pediatric audiology. Being accepted into this program was a dream come true.

I used a personal FM system in all my classes at Akron. In addition, I was able to supplement my own notes with the help of a classmate who took notes on carbon copy notepaper. At the end of each lecture, she would give me a copy.

In my second week of graduate studies, the professors asked the students to begin assessing patients' hearing in the audiology clinic. I asked my patients to wear my FM transmitter during their hearing tests. The transmitter helped me hear their responses clearly during speech discrimination tests. During Auditory-Verbal sessions with my children, I used the FM system as well, with the child wearing the transmitter. Not only was this "crutch" critical for my listening and spoken language development, it also proved critical for my job.

After two years of hard work at Akron, I received my M.A. in audiology. I passed the American Speech-Language-Hearing Association (ASHA) certification exam and began preparing my application to practice in Ontario. I returned home the day after I graduated.

Martin and I were married in 1996, on Labor Day. It was hot and sunny, and we were deliriously happy. We began our married life in a tiny house in a small town north of Toronto. Martin returned to school and I set out to look for a job.

Job hunting brought back my old insecurities. The positions advertised in the paper were like the boys I contemplated chasing in high school. In this case, the jobs just seemed to want to run away from me. Doubts about my ability to do well in the workplace because of my hearing loss began to resurface, and I even wondered if I was unmarketable with hearing aids. Martin did his best to be reassuring, by reminding me that my perfect job was not yet out there.

It turned out that Martin was right. Nearly a year from the day I graduated, I managed to secure a position as a clinical audiologist at an occupational health clinic in Toronto. Shortly thereafter, I was offered the job of my dreams as an Auditory-Verbal therapist at the Learning to Listen Foundation (LTLF). The supervisor at the occupational health clinic asked me to stay on for work in the evenings and I immediately accepted the offer. For two years, I worked during the day at the LTLF, and two evenings a week I worked at the audiology clinic. It was perfect.

Back in Familiar Water

For 15 years, I had successfully sailed unknown waters, but now, with the Learning to Listen Foundation, I had returned home. I was better equipped, with a more refined set of skills and abilities, all essential as I faced what would be the most challenging and rewarding job I have ever known. As my mentor, and as director of the LTLF's Auditory Learning Centre, Warren expected my best efforts. He treated me as he would any other therapist: with kindness, honesty, and respect.

The best part about my work at LTLF is that I share in the joy of helping parents give their children the gift of listening and spoken language, a gift given to me by my own parents.

Many in my family say that my speech has improved since working at LTLF. Perhaps it is the heightened awareness of the need to be clear and concise when communicating with children and their parents. I do know I've become a better listener. I continue to use the FM system for Auditory-Verbal sessions, conferences, and staff meetings.

In recent years, the staff at LTLF has grown. Each colleague has taught me something new, and I cherish these learning opportunities. Most important, I've been fortunate to work as a team member with many extremely talented therapists. I continue to be amazed by the power of teamwork among caring Auditory-Verbal therapists and other professionals.

Often I am moved to tears by the accomplishments of children with whom I work. Hearing technology has made it easier for children to hear and learn spoken language through listening. Children are reaching age-appropriate speech and language skills in half the time it took my generation. The dedication of parents and family members to their children continues to thrill me, and I am reminded of my mother's hard work and the tears of joy she experienced when I finally achieved a skill that had taken me so long to learn.

My Life Today

My return to LTLF has brought Martin and me the gift of new lifelong friendships. For example, through Warren, I met Jonathan Samson — the first person I had met with a positive attitude about his hearing loss. He was a breath of fresh air. He seemed to have every assistive listening device gadget on the market. I was also impressed with his level of independence, and I applaud his parents for how they helped him become the person he is. Martin and I enjoyed watching him gain even more independence with his cochlear implant and shared in the joys of his new auditory potential.

Jonathan introduced us to John Humphreys, who also has a positive attitude about his hearing loss. Most impressive is his capacity for joy and kindness to others. Martin and I gravitated toward his wonderful qualities and are proud to call him one of our closest friends.

The best part of a circle of friends is when it continues to grow. Jonathan met and married his wife Tania, and they have a darling little boy named Jacob. John soon met Andrea. Perhaps, to some degree, we are friends because we share a common bond of deafness, but we are friends foremost because we share common interests and values.

Martin and I were thrilled when we found out we were expecting our own baby in March of 2001. But we never expected the elation we felt during the ultrasound when we heard Emily's heartbeat for the first time. I was overcome not only with the emotion of hearing that she actually existed, but also by the enormity of realizing how close I had come to missing out on this incredible experience had my parents accepted that initial prognosis

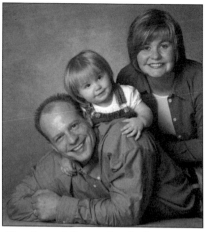

Martin and I were elated when we heard Emily's heartbeat for the first time. I was overcome by the enormity of realizing how close I came to missing out on this incredible experience.

when my hearing loss was diagnosed. More precious was hearing her first cries when she was born, and then hearing her cries subside as soon as she heard my voice. My mother was there with us for that magical moment.

Emily is 3 years old and the apple of our eyes. She was a very good baby, always able to sleep through the night — a trait she inherited from her father. She never misses a meal — a trait she inherited from me. And she enjoys life — a trait she inherited from both of us. Her hearing is within normal limits, and Martin and I are working hard to teach her English and German.

Hopes and dreams will continue to grow. That is the beauty of life . . . it is ever-changing and bountiful in its gifts if you choose to accept them. My hearing loss was a gift that I chose to accept. I am grateful for the opportunities it has given me.

Hopes, Dreams, and Guidance

In conclusion, I offer the following words of hope and encouragement for all who read these stories, so they may help make the world a better place for those of us who are deaf or hard of hearing:

> Creatively overcome obstacles,
> Have heroes as role models,
> Inspire others with your example,
> Listen to your heart,
> Develop relationships through the language of possibilities,
> Respect those who give honest and constructive feedback,
> Earn opportunities, don't expect them,
> Never give up.

CHAPTER 3

John-David Humphreys

The supreme happiness of life is the conviction that we are loved.

— Victor Hugo

I WAS BORN ON A BRIGHT SEPTEMBER AFTERNOON IN 1970, MY PARENTS' ONLY CHILD. I was a healthy and happy baby, visually very alert. It was quickly apparent, though, that I wasn't making the babbling sounds typical of an infant with normal hearing. For example, when my parents called my name or closed a door behind me, they noticed that I showed no response. Gradually, I was examined by a variety of specialists and a number of theories were postulated. One psychologist confirmed that my cognitive abilities were intact, but suggested I have my hearing tested. That clinched it for my parents.

When I was finally diagnosed at 20 months with a profound bilateral sensorineural hearing loss, I immediately began auditory training — the process by which a child with hearing loss learns to listen and speak using a specific curriculum and assistive devices such as hearing aids or a cochlear implant. Auditory training is predicated on the reality that, unlike children with normal hearing, those who are deaf are highly unlikely to acquire acoustic integrity and verbal skills without early diagnosis and intervention.

In Good Hands

My first teacher was Louise Crawford, a renowned expert in Auditory-Verbal therapy with a vast repertoire of experience and skills. I had lessons with her once a week for seven years.

One of my parents' first questions upon meeting her was how long therapy would last. They thought it would be a period of merely a few weeks, only to have her tell them it would likely be seven or eight years. My family recognized the value of perseverance, which is a most important factor in the entire therapeutic process. When all prospects seem dark, dreary, and dim (perhaps because the child is less than forthcoming in responding to auditory stimuli), it usually is sheer, dogged perseverance that carries the day. Even with the most sophisticated technologies, the acquisition of language will still take time. Although we anticipated a long period of learning, my parents adopted the philosophy that it is not the length of the symphony, but the quality of the music that ultimately matters. Little did my parents and I know then that during therapy we would be introduced to a "symphony" that would exceed our grandest expectations.

With the passage of time, my lessons with Louise progressed from simple auditory stimulation (i.e., the cow says "moo"; the airplane says "ahhh"; "bu, bu, bu" says the bus) to my first word — "meow," which overjoyed my parents as it was concrete evidence that therapy was working — and then to more complex sounds such as the distinction between "ch" in church and "ch" in machine. I am still learning language to this day and recently discovered, for instance, that the famed Champs-Elysées in Paris is pronounced quite differently from how it reads.

My early auditory stimulation reminds me of the line in the A.A. Milne classic *Winnie the Pooh:* "I am a Bear of Very Little Brain, and long words Bother me." Simultaneous to my auditory stimulation, Louise endeavored to help me develop a robust vocabulary, a refined command of language, a fulgent imagination, and an ability to read and write with vigor, courage, and excellence. Her personal qualities of great wisdom, impeccable integrity, and deep kindness are what I value most. She has received the highest honor that our country can bestow — the Order of Canada — for her work with children who are deaf.

'Everything in its own Time'

The therapist has both longitudinal and latitudinal experience — longitudinal in that he or she is with the child for several years and assumes the persona of a close family member; latitudinal because of the breadth of his or her experience in dealing with many styles of learning and many personality types. The longitudinal viewpoint allows the therapist to devise long-term plans, to analyse the child's progress, and to tailor therapeutic strategies accordingly. Latitudinal observation, on the other hand, focuses on specific milestones set by the therapist on the child's road to spoken language.

Each child is different, however. Although the pace of my progress varied during therapy, Louise was quick to affirm the age-old adage, "Everything in its own time."

Still, the primary client in Auditory-Verbal therapy is the parent, not the child. Therapists guide parents in teaching their children — a "guide on the side," as Warren Estabrooks likes to say. Adapting the goals established in each lesson, the parents must use every available waking hour to help their child attain his or her maximum auditory and linguistic potential.

Every evening when they came home from work, my parents conducted lessons to teach me how to listen and speak. I occasionally resisted these lessons, simply because I was interested in doing something else, such as playing with my friends. When I wandered off, however, my mother would begin teaching Boody, my teddy bear. Of course, that piqued my curiosity and I would return to join the exercise. My friends would sometimes come over for the lessons with my parents since they found it such a novel and exciting experience. As I reflect on this, it was a most astute practice in that it made my friends aware that they needed to speak clearly and adopt alternative strategies if I misunderstood something.

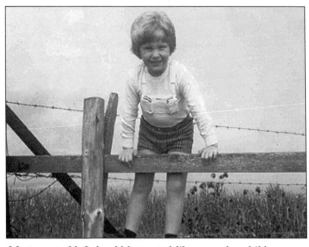

My parents felt I should be treated like any other child.

Certain words are, by nature, very easy to explain to children (e.g., most nouns and verbs); however, other words or idioms and abstract concepts tend to be quite complex. In teaching me the word *beautiful*, for example, my mother showed me a number of pictures we have in our home. There is a painting titled "The Doctor" by Sir Luke Fildes, which is housed in the Tate Gallery in London. It depicts a distinguished-looking doctor ministering to an impoverished and gravely ill child as her grieving parents look on. My mother used this to express the beauty of compassion, mercy, and kindness. We also have a painting of a mother tending to her children, which my mother used to teach me the beauty of a parent's love. And, to demonstrate the beauty of dedication, work, and perseverance, my mother showed me a picture of harvesters reaping wheat in the fields of France.

The word *consent* is another important abstract. I learned that my teachers needed my parents' consent for me to go on a school trip, and that my pediatrician needed their consent to give me a vaccination. So, when I next saw my pediatrician, I asked him, "Are you going to give me an injection today?" He wondered why I was asking, to which I responded, "Because if you are, you need my mommy's consent." Startled, he remarked that I was quite precocious. Observing his demeanor, I replied with an idiom I had recently learned — "Don't get your knickers in a twist" — which broke him up with laughter.

Both my parents continued to work full time as I grew up, notwithstanding the advice of some experts who say at least one parent should consider remaining at home. Neither of them took any unusual steps in the process of teaching me to listen and speak, apart from our regular evening lessons. They felt I should be treated like any other child. Then, as now, I was constantly aware of their deep, deep love for me.

Many parents with whom I have spoken have been interested in the fact that our family has never owned a television set. My parents considered purchasing one when I was young, but Louise wisely advised them that it would distract me from my lessons.

Foreign Exchange

The effectiveness of the Auditory-Verbal approach cannot be overstated. For example, when I was 12, I began corresponding with a boy in Germany who was hearing-impaired. In one of my letters, I indicated rather nonchalantly that I would like to visit Germany some day. His family very kindly invited my family to stay with them for a month on their farm in the Bavarian hinterland. The exquisite scenery was beyond description. My German friend and his younger brother are both deaf. When their family met us, they were astonished that I was able to listen and speak; they thought, perhaps, that my hearing loss was not as severe as that of their children. They arranged to have my hearing tested at one of their clinics and were amazed to find by comparing our audiograms that my hearing loss was, in fact, greater than their sons'. I spent some time at German teaching facilities for children who are deaf and, in retrospect, remain quite impressed with the quality of those facilities and the education they delivered. Unfortunately, Auditory-Verbal therapy had yet to be introduced in their country.

One area in which many families find it a struggle to persevere is in the number of visits made to hearing aid dealers for repairs and other unanticipated events (such as broken parts or outgrown earmolds). These issues are less pressing today because of the durability of most devices on the market. Sudden and unanticipated events can be especially challenging when one travels. Once when I was in England, my hearing aid recharger refused to work. Fortunately, our family knew an elderly gentleman there who made watches as a hobby and had been an electronics expert during World War II. He was able to locate the problem and fix it. The alternative would have been to attempt to locate a hearing aid dealer in London, not unlike searching for a needle in a haystack.

When I was a small boy, my mother and I met a group of gentlemen in navy blazers and gray trousers near our home in Toronto. I went up to them and began trying on their hats. One gentleman with a handlebar mustache approached my mother and explained that they were the "Dambusters," the famed group of Allied fighter pilots from World War II. They were in town for a reunion. My mother explained to them that I had been diagnosed as profoundly deaf just a few weeks before. The gentleman whispered to my mother in kind tones: "I will pray for your son."

A Special Friendship

One of the outstanding gifts of my childhood was the commencement of a lifelong friendship with Jonathan Samson. Jonathan and I were both diagnosed the same week in 1972. We have spent countless days and weekends together. I remember being exposed to his Jewish faith very early and remember watching his father bless the children at the beginning of each Sabbath.

Jonathan and I sometimes had difficulty understanding each other on the telephone. He would suggest that we meet at a certain place at a certain time, and I thought he was saying something along the lines of: "I've decided to take up golf." Or, he would say: "Let's meet at 1," and I would say, "No, let's meet at 1." Then he would say, "That's right, 1," to which I would respond, "Not 5, but 1."

I had the great joy and honor of participating in Jonathan's wedding just 100 yards from Westminster Abbey in London, England. As I will describe below, Jonathan and his wife Tania were instrumental in introducing me to the wonderful woman I love.

As I reflect on my experiences, I am deeply moved. The road down which I've journeyed has been hedged in by a plethora of wonders. One source of enormous fulfilment is sharing the reality that children who are deaf have a great deal of hope, and that there is a network of people willing to nurture, befriend, and guide them and their parents.

Coming of Age

It was a beautiful Indian summer morning . . . bright, cool, and crisp — and it was my first day at school. I remember it vividly, almost as though it were yesterday. My parents never gave a thought to the possibility of sending me away from home to a school for the deaf. For them, as for most parents, the very idea of separation was unbearable. Children need their parents. Love, affection, and bonding with one's family becomes even more significant for children who are deaf.

My parents gave some thought to having me attend a private school in Toronto, but Louise candidly advised them to send me to a school "where the teachers are kind."

Early exposure to the academic mainstream equips the child who is deaf with lifelong skills. There are many experiences with which the child must contend, as well as the countless whims, mores, and vicissitudes, all comprising the complex mosaic of the "hearing" world. In primary school, I asked many rhetorical questions: "Why am I selected last on the team?" "What will I do if a friend makes a joke and I respond inappropriately?" "Why am I deaf?" The classroom and the schoolyard proved to be tremendous training grounds for the great playing field of life. Real life molds, shapes, and hones.

I always attended a public school and was always in a regular class. The only distinction between me and my peers was the regular itinerant assistance I received. High quality itinerant assistance is something that every parent of a child with hearing loss should take advantage of — its merits can never be underestimated. I was extremely fortunate to have the caliber of itinerant teachers that I did.

The school teachers I remember best are those who had great creative prowess and the ability to keep their students motivated and interested in the topics at bar. Some aspects of grade school were awkward, such as learning from films (there was no possible way to understand the narrators). Moreover, given the great diligence required in mastering English, the study of other languages (from the auditory, enunciation, and verbal perspectives) wasn't easy.

Middle school was more complicated than grade school. I attribute this to the fact that in grade school everyone who grew up with me knew "who and what I was all about," so they generally didn't view me as overly different. Middle school, however, was a melting pot of children from all backgrounds, most of whom had never met a person who was deaf before. I was singled out for occasional teasing.

One instance proved to be somewhat embarrassing. All of the students in my grade and those from several other schools went to Toronto's Young People's Theatre to view the play *Of Mice and Men*. Before the curtains were lifted, the crowd (naturally) chattered excitedly. My teacher had just finished chastising another teacher for seating me in the balcony, where I would be unable to read the actors' lips. She insisted that I sit near the front, and I was relocated. Perhaps emboldened by her success in this matter, she then went to the front of the auditorium, raised her arms, and asked for silence. Pointing toward me, she proceeded to advise the audience that "John Humphreys, over there, is profoundly deaf and will be unable to hear the play if you continue to make such noise. I insist that you remain silent." Her intentions, at least, were noble.

There were some rare instances when a teacher refused to wear the FM transmitter or showed little compassion or interest in understanding the communication challenges facing a student with hearing loss. When I related various events of this nature to my parents, they gave me wise and loving counsel about conducting myself with diplomacy, dignity, and grace. I learned early how to stand on my own feet. If the gravity of the situation demanded it, my parents would act as advocates, but those occasions were few and far between. Essentially, I learned about advocating for myself, and for others. I strongly encourage parents of children who are deaf to resist the urge to plunge into the fray at every turn, so their children can learn how to carry themselves with tact and aplomb. There will be those times when a child does need a champion at the gates. If so, I recommend that parents partner with their child's itinerant teacher to pursue appropriate avenues of redress. The itinerant teacher offers a thorough understanding of the school system, coupled with a great deal of experience.

High School Memories

My high school, Leaside High in Toronto, was splendid, and offered a group of marvelous teachers. There was a very clear expectation that students would be exposed to a pulsating variety of experiences and that work of the highest quality was the norm. A premium was placed on excellent reading, writing, and oratory skills. To quote Francis Bacon: "Reading maketh a full man, conference a ready man, and writing an exact man."

It occasionally took time for my teachers to learn how to engage me with comfort and ease. My wonderful French teacher would explain the intricacies of the French language while standing inches in front of me as I sat. Evidently, she wanted to ensure that I fully understood all those intonations of which any Parisienne would be proud. She would lean forward as she spoke, and I would lean forward, too. I eventually apprised my mother of this circumstance, and when my mother suggested that I tell her the FM system was sufficient, I exclaimed: "But, I like it!"

I did well in high school, which I attribute to those teachers who had the insight to recognize that my hearing loss was a vital part of my make-up and who drew out my various strengths in that context. To their great credit, my teachers did not accord me any preferential treatment — in fact, I sometimes think they were more demanding because I was deaf. This, combined with the erudition, savvy, and perceptiveness of my itinerant teacher Ross Fletcher invigorated me for the tasks set before me.

During my high school summers, I discovered the joys of working at Camp Ahmek, a camp for boys in Algonquin Park, Ontario. I was a counselor-in-training for one summer, and a camp counselor for two more. As part of my responsibilities, I had the bliss of leading my campers on canoe trips into the wilderness. Several years before, a friend of mine had taken me on a canoe trip through Algonquin Park and I became quickly enchanted. The camp offered fantastic opportunities to learn and teach various sports, including horseback riding, sailing, and canoeing. I also met a wonderful group of people, some of whom I have stayed in touch with to this day. Around the campfire at night, it was difficult for me to follow others in conversation, so I often volunteered to tell stories, which meant I could control the ebb and flow.

University Accomplishments

In the fall of 1989, I commenced a joint specialist degree in history and political science at the University of Toronto. This is unusual, I'm told, as most students who are deaf tend to focus on mathematics and the sciences. When I discussed my choices with a reliable authority, I was dismayed to discover that 80% of students who are deaf graduate from high school with a fourth-grade reading level. Heartbreaking! Those of us who have learned to listen and speak have an obligation to espouse the virtues of Auditory-Verbal therapy when and where we can.

Before the first class of any course I took, I met with the professor to explain the nature of my hearing loss and ask whether he or she would wear the FM system while lecturing. I also asked if the professor would announce during the first lecture that there was a student with hearing loss in the class who would greatly appreciate the help of volunteer notetakers. This was fantastic because it gave me the luxury of making some splendid friends.

In one history class, the professor hadn't met me yet, but was aware that I was in his class. He called out, "Who's the deaf student?" He looked at a very quiet, shy sort of fellow a few rows back and said with an avuncular smile, "It's you, isn't it?" I raised my hand and said, "Actually, it's me, sir." He was astonished, and blurted, "But, you can't be deaf!" I assured him that I was. Evidently he didn't realize that one could be deaf and yet listen and speak at the same time.

I graduated from the University of Toronto with high distinction, earning my honors bachelor of arts. One evening, I came home to find my mother bursting with excitement to relay the news that I was the Victoria College gold medalist in political economy, a fascinating branch of political science.

During my undergraduate years, I had considered a host of possible venues that I was interested in pursuing: the ministry, business, international relations, psychology, teaching children who are deaf, politics, and law. The doors opened into law. For the duration of my undergraduate studies and my first year of law school, I had relied on the notes prepared by my classmates. Unfortunately, there is no way to accurately gauge the quality of another student's notes. Given the demand for precision in language in law, and given the abundance of linguistic acrobatics and semantic subtleties, I felt it would be astute to try real-time captioning. A captionist would come to each class and type verbatim what the professor was saying. He or she would bring a laptop computer, which enabled me to read while the professor spoke. Once the notes were edited, I received a hard copy.

There are some drawbacks to captioning: (a) the quality of the captioning varies from captionist to captionist; (b) captioning does not capture inflections or intonations (which makes it very difficult to know on which points a speaker has placed particular emphasis); and (c) unlike handwritten notes, captioned notes are not organized; rather, they are seamless and run without interruption. Accordingly, I recommend that captioning be used as an adjunct to handwritten notes so they can be contrasted against each other.

When I graduated from Osgoode Hall Law School in Toronto, I attained the highest standing in my class in international law.

Acoustic Aberrations

In my final year of university, I lost my residual hearing in the space of 20 minutes. Initially, I was convinced that it was simply battery drainage in my hearing aids. When I tried several spare hearing aids, however, I reached the daunting conclusion that it was, in fact, my hearing. The specialists I consulted were mystified. One doctor postulated that it was an illusory respiratory virus that I contracted while traveling in the Middle East the previous summer.

Because of the remarkably high quality of therapy and itinerant services I had received — and especially the guidance of my parents — I had attained unusual auditory acuity. Telephones, for example, posed few problems. Indeed, in many cases, I was able to recognize callers just by listening to their voices.

When I lost my residual hearing, however, I became totally dependent on lipreading and relied on others to help me with telephone conversations. What a dreary existence. In the practice of law, rapid and accurate communication is essential. In a more Utopian society, clients and colleagues would have the time, patience, and inclination to render the requisite assistance to communicate freely and fluidly.

The Implant Alternative

For some time, I had been hearing of the marvels of the cochlear implant. Then my friend Jonathan took the courageous step of opting for implant surgery. He researched the materials and canvassed the field with characteristic assiduity. The proof of the pudding, though, lay in the impact the implant had on his life. In February, 1998, I was visiting Jonathan when he turned suddenly in response to a sound that I did not hear. His mother asked me, "Did you hear that?" I was amazed.

Soon after Jonathan's surgery, another good friend of mine, Sol Fried, also opted for an implant. No longer could I consider this a remote option. Ever since I had lost my residual hearing, my parents and Louise had urged me to consider the surgery, but I rather stubbornly refused. They continued to prod me. Then it was Jonathan, and eventually Sol. Their parents, too, urged me to take the leap. Finally, one morning in the early spring of 1998, I decided that I would go for tests to determine my eligibility for an implant. The rest is history.

> ## Something deeply hidden had to be behind things.
> – *Albert Einstein*

One of my chief concerns was whether I would be able to receive postimplant therapy. Louise and my previous teachers had kindly offered to provide therapy; however, I felt that it would be unfair to accept their services and deprive them of their leisure time. They would be the first to deny any such inconvenience, but I felt awkward nevertheless. In the weeks leading up to surgery, I became increasingly concerned, given my knowledge that therapy is vital to the successful application of the implant. Jonathan suggested that I apply to the Learning to Listen Foundation.

The board of directors of the foundation very graciously adopted a policy of embracing adults as space permits. You can imagine my joy! Among other policies and criteria that must be met, the chief criterion is that the client be willing to undergo the rigors of therapy with a flexible spirit and a true desire to benefit.

Besides Warren Estabrooks, director of the LTLF's Auditory Learning Centre, another LTLF therapist, Karen MacIver-Lux, provided great encouragement and support in the decision-making process. It was wonderful to have someone my own age who could speak from the perspective of both a professional and a friend. Karen has a crystal clear understanding of the interplay between audiological perception and Auditory-Verbal application.

Shortly before my surgery, Warren interviewed me at length. He was extremely careful to set out the expectations of both therapist and client. Expectations were vital to ensure a therapeutic paradigm within which the principals in this process could maneuver.

The surgical aspect of the implant is very straightforward. Granted, results can vary widely, but in the hands of a first-rate professional team, it is hard to go far wrong. Such was my team at Sunnybrook Hospital in Toronto.

My surgeon, Julian Nedzelski, is a man who exudes great confidence, has a wealth of experience and wide repute, and has kindness tempered by much common sense and sagacity. My audiologists, Amy Ng and David Shipp, are also professionals of the highest caliber.

A few days before the surgery, I was challenged to consider changing my "ear of implant." I had decided on my left as I believed that I had nothing to lose; however, there was the possibility that my right ear — with its history of acoustic stimulation — would prove a more beneficial site. Jonathan urged me to correspond on this with Dr. Noel Cohen in New York. Dr. Cohen wrote back immediately, reassuring me that there was no consensus as to whether the "good" or the "bad" ear should be implanted. I consulted with Warren again and am grateful that he had the integrity to urge me to explore unknowns — I chose the left ear. As Victor Hugo once wrote: "Great perils have this beauty, that they bring to light the fraternity of strangers."

'He Maketh the Deaf to Hear'

The surgery was, of course, technical. Pain was kept to a minimum. In the preparation room, however, I was asked to change into a blue, ill-fitting hospital gown. The nurse came by with a pair of white stockings and asked me to wear them. I was quite pleased since I thought it would keep my legs a little warmer and afford some modesty; however, I suggested to the nurse that my shorts would accomplish the task equally well. She replied, "But Mr. Humphreys, these are constriction stockings, and because you are having bowel surgery you are required to wear them." Can you imagine if someone else woke up with a cochlear implant!

Five weeks later, the great day came for activating my implant. I felt no nervousness or trepidation — rather, trenchant curiosity. David Shipp and I went through the activation process alone. This is good practice, since a client might be tempted to respond differently in the presence of a loved one. That is, when asked whether you are hearing something or are comfortable, the tendency is to be more upbeat than honest when someone you don't want to worry is nearby (at least in my case). I wanted the first words I heard to be special, so I asked David to read from the Gospel of Mark in the King James Bible:

> He hath done all things well;
> He maketh the deaf to hear.

David read solemnly and sweetly. I went to meet my mother and we shared some moments of exquisite tenderness.

The implant was on. It was a series of vibrations. I felt as though I was "feeling" sounds rather than hearing them. Following Warren's guidance, my mother took me for a walk to hear different sounds in my neighborhood. Cars and buses I could barely hear at all. Running water was absolutely horrid, as were dishes clanging. From time to time, I would turn the speech processor off (as I still do) to appreciate the true meaning of "Silence is

Golden." That evening, I visited Louise and she performed a simple test, although I was unable to answer appropriately. With constant good cheer, however, she encouraged me to persevere.

As I reflect on the "buzz" of sounds, I'm reminded of the words of W. B. Yeats:

> I will arise and go now, and go to Innisfree,
> And a small cabin build there, of clay and wattles made:
> Nine bean-rows will I have there, a hive for the honeybee,
> And live alone in the bee-loud glade.

My experience was, in every sense, a "bee-loud glade"! As our family knows, Innisfree is a place of calm repose, and that is where the road was to lead me.

I began therapy and it proved to be a process filled with excitement and pleasure. One of my parents almost always attended the session with me to record how they might continue therapy at home. Friends of mine have attended as well. We began with some very simple techniques and a process known as priming. Essentially, priming is designed to draw the client into listening. Basic priming is: "John?" along with the response, "Yes, Warren?" Examples of intermediate priming are: "Can you hear me?" . . . "Are you listening?" . . . "Are you ready?" A secondary priming example is: "I'm going to do letters of the alphabet now," or "I'm going to give you some spondee words," referring to two-syllable words that have equal stress on each syllable. Complex priming comprises a rapid series of questions or comments, often unrelated, embodying complex ideas.

Once I was "primed," we launched into specific exercises. At the beginning of the journey, we did a few very basic things:

- ❧ The Ling Six-Sound Test (ah, oo, ee, sh, s, and m);
- ❧ Words with one syllable, two syllables, three syllables, etc. — my task being to select the right number of syllables in a word; and
- ❧ Simple questions: "When's your birthday?"; "What is your telephone number and your e-mail address?"

As therapy progressed, we moved on to closed-set words and spondee words. Closed-set words are words that one does not recognize immediately; however, within the context of the set (i.e., colors, animals, capital cities) one can make an educated deduction.

In the meantime, my parents continued to work with me at home. It was always exciting, interesting, and deeply moving — "moving" in the sense that I was living my childhood once again. This was wonderful in that it made me keenly aware of the sacrifices and sheer determination of the families, teachers, and therapists of children who are deaf. My mother has great skill in conveying words and concepts, and my father has stayed up late many evenings singing with me. Since he sings so beautifully and with such

> My parents continued to work with me at home. It was always deeply moving in the sense that I was living my childhood once again.

passion, that has been particularly lovely. Both my parents are natural conversationalists, and both have a remarkable sense of grandeur and wonder. Love, combined with wonder, is the imprimatur graven on the heart of the child with fine parents.

Amy Ng, one of my audiologists, often made adjustments to the implant to fine-tune my hearing as much as possible. I put my old hearing aid out of sight and disciplined myself not to touch it. I can assure you that in the first days the temptation was very strong.

In any event, I progressed in therapy to numbers and letters of the alphabet. I was given three chances at word recognition. We also used the strategies of spelling the word or using it in a meaningful sentence. This makes the information more acoustically salient. The therapists at LTLF are highly skilled at leading the client to recognition by a process of conceptual reasoning. That is, rather than spelling a word or using it in a sentence, they would bring in similar, but not identical, ideas. For example, if one struggles over the name "Tokyo," the therapist will mention Mount Fuji, bonsai, etc., with no direct clues. This is excellent therapy because it lodges a vast repertoire of language in the client's auditory-memory cortex. Moreover, its more difficult nature tends to stroke the client's mind all the more.

Single numbers were difficult since so many sound alike. One, nine, and ten each have the nasal "n"; two and three, five and nine have similar-sounding vowels; and four and five, depending on the speaker, can be alike depending on the strength of the "f" sound. One can only imagine the difficulties incumbent on the mastery of letters. Even now, letters are tricky for me.

Eventually, I progressed to open-set words (i.e., words with no context), to singing, and eventually to interactive conversation. Some therapy sessions have been solely conversation-based. This is the summit view of therapy as it most closely resembles natural communication.

Other exercises included the use of the telephone and the mastery of conversation from a distance or with background noise.

Although the pinnacle of therapy is seamless and interesting conversation, the most challenging aspect of therapy is the recognition of single-syllable words, which are, under the rules of acoustic science, extremely difficult to master. As examples:

> pen, men, pin, pan, man, Nan
>
> soap (the "p" is not sounded)
>
> coin (really sounds like two syllables)
>
> boy, bore, more (which sound alike)

I continue to be delighted by surprises. Not long ago, I was riding in a car, reading various work-related documents. The radio was crackling loudly. It suddenly occurred to me that I subconsciously understood the newscaster despite concentrating on other matters.

Therapeutic Excellence

Some elements of therapy have been especially helpful. As one may expect, auditory mistakes are rampant. Warren and Karen have been wonderful friends. They have worked assiduously to understand the cause of an acoustic error. They would encourage me when the error was a good one, and would explain the science behind certain words and concepts and why they could be particularly difficult to grasp. Warren would also be careful not to praise when it was inappropriate. Therapy is robust, varied, and fast-paced, and it can be exhausting. A major advantage in the process, however, is that the client's mind is constantly piqued. Fast-paced therapy allows breadth to become breadth and depth. I have seen how skillful the therapist must be. The therapist must be adaptable to meet the needs of very complex people in a very complex world. He or she must keep abreast of technology, medicine, and education to maintain the cachet of their practice.

I wrote earlier about how the parent is the true client in childhood therapy. In adult therapy, the client was me. This is a very unusual situation since it yields to diagnostics, prognosis, and treatment being in the hands of both the therapist and client. The therapist guides and recommends, but the client decides and tweaks.

Throughout this process, I have often been asked if I did the right thing. I have absolutely no regrets, but I will say that despite "better" hearing — in the sense that it is broader and more acute, which I enjoy — it took a while to arrive at the same sweetness or fidelity of sound that my hearing aids afforded. I tried the hearing aid on a while after my implant and found it was far inferior in both acuity and timbre. Wonderfully, music is now even more beautiful than it once was. When I first had my implant, the descriptive analogy I used was that the implant allowed me to read more (as in *The Economist* or *The New Yorker*); however, it had only the black and white of those two journals rather than the many hues of a Ladybird book that I enjoyed with my hearing aids. Over time, though, the colors began to filter in — blues, violets, magentas, greens, and golds of every hue.

I'm rather fond of the following from *The Wind in the Willows*:

> With a smile of much happiness on his face, and something of a listening look still lingering there, the weary Rat was fast asleep.

Traveling Man

Since I was very young, I have been enchanted by travel. I attribute this to the many trips we took as a family, or I with just my father, to all those magnificent and mysterious places around the world. My parents had the wonderful gift of making each adventure precisely that — an adventure. Although I am biased, my father is a teller of stories *par excellence*. He has journeyed throughout the world, and his tales of distant climes have always enthralled me.

One day, when I was in 10th grade, I was looking for something to read and began to roam the halls of my library. On the spine of a certain book was a title that caught my eye: "So You Want to Work on a Kibbutz?" I had absolutely no idea what a kibbutz was, so I signed the book out and read it. I was riveted, and decided that that was precisely what I would like to do. And so I did. At the end of my third year at the University of Toronto, I visited Israel and worked on a kibbutz for two months. (A note about kibbutzim. Hart and Renata, good friends of Jonathan, Karen, and me, met on a kibbutz and subsequently married. Neither Hart nor Renata is deaf; however, they exemplify the type of friendship a person with hearing loss would enjoy. They know to speak clearly and logically. They never dilute the intellect of the substance under discussion. They are fun, engaging, understanding, and stalwarts.)

While in Israel, I also traveled to various parts of the country. I slept by the Dead Sea, climbed Masada in the stillness of the night just before sunrise, and crossed the Sinai into Egypt and explored Cairo. I then returned to Israel to tour Jerusalem and Tel Aviv, and ventured through the Golan.

It was supremely enchanting to meet different people with different life experiences. Two incidents in Israel leap to mind. The first involves a border crossing from Israel into the Sinai. At the back of the coach were two fellow travelers who knew only sign language. They were greatly distressed because they had no way of communicating with anyone or understanding anything being said to them. I was struck, very forcibly, by the fact they were in such an isolated position. The second incident was my own experience of isolation. I needed to make telephone calls to my parents to discuss the various university courses I would be taking in the fall. I asked someone to be an interpreter for me. It was an extremely difficult process since the interpreter's English was not perfect and I simply couldn't understand what my parents were saying. My mother has commented more than once on the great turmoil she has felt whenever I was a great distance from home and she was unable to converse with me normally on the telephone.

> My mother felt great turmoil whenever I was far from home and she was unable to converse with me normally on the telephone.

On another occasion, I read an article about horseracing in Mongolia and decided that I would like to visit that part of the world. Originally, I was going to spend two months solely in Mongolia; however, I decided to cast my net a little further afield. I began my journey in Singapore, which was of great significance to me since my grandfather had been a prisoner of war in World War II. I then traveled up to Malaysia and into Thailand. I flew to Hong Kong and from there sailed to Guangzhou (formerly Canton). I traveled through inland China up to Beijing and on to Mongolia (my original destination, and a fascinating country). My next destination was the far west of China, namely, Urumqi (pronounced Urumchee) and Kashgar, on the old Silk Road. My ultimate goal from there was to travel into Pakistan along the Karakoram Highway (which is the highest highway in the world) and down to Islamabad/Rawalpindi. I then flew to Karachi, back to Singapore, and on to England.

People have often asked me which area was my favorite. This is difficult to say since there were so many beautiful spots. I must say, however, that Singapore has a certain appealing exoticism and the Karakorams were breathtaking in their scenery and in the warmth of their people, all juxtaposed against the wild and rugged remoteness of their land.

There are a few tales of that trip worth relating. When I was in Kuala Lumpur, the capital city of peninsular Malaysia, I met a gentleman who insisted on taking me on the back of his motorcycle throughout the city to meet his friends and family. In the end, he offered me presents to carry home. When I asked why he was being so kind, he simply said, "Because you cannot hear." This was tremendously humbling and moving.

By the time I reached Hong Kong, I was feeling a little lonely, being miles from anyone I knew and unable to chat with anybody or simply to pick up the phone and call my family. So, remembering a beautiful story I once read about the ability of fragrances to evoke memories, I went to a shop and found a perfume my mother often wears. I sprayed a little bit on a card and carried it around in my wallet. The delicious fragrance brought many lovely images to mind.

On the train from Guangzhou to Beijing (two days and two nights nonstop, with very minimal facilities) I met a man who was extremely interested in my hearing loss and insisted it could be cured using a method a professor friend of his had developed called Qi Gong. Needless to say, I advised him that I would stick with my hearing aids for the time being.

In Mongolia, I met an elderly gentleman with hearing aids. I asked if I could test his battery and found that it had drained. When I asked, through the Mongolian/English interpreter, how often they changed batteries (which usually needs to be done every week), I was told that he was using the same batteries he was given when he bought the hearing aid two years earlier. The luxuries of the West were sadly lacking there.

Interestingly, I met a large group of young people who were deaf in Ulaan Baator, Mongolia's capital. They knew only sign language and clamored excitedly when the sign language interpreter explained that I was also deaf but that I could speak. They wanted to know how it was possible. Hopefully, some day, programs to enable individuals who are deaf to listen and speak can be delivered to the farthest reaches of the earth.

I had a similar experience on a subsequent trip to Thailand. I was in the deep south of Thailand, near the Malaysian border, when I met another group of young people who were deaf. They, too, were amazed that I was able to speak. I shall never forget the look of deep yearning and longing I saw in their eyes to be in my place. One of them placed his hand on my throat to feel my muscles as I spoke and was able to utter a surprisingly similar sound on that basis alone.

Even in countries that are considered highly westernized, such as the United Kingdom, Israel, Japan, New Zealand, Singapore, and even Canada, many people have told me they were amazed that I could listen and speak.

A Career in Law

I practice law for a living and usually describe myself as a business lawyer with a hybrid background in securities and corporate finance, the emphasis being on securities law. I have also practiced not-for-profit law and have worked with clients on matters of Estates and private business.

At present, I am a Crown Attorney with the Ontario Securities Commission. My particular branch investigates and prosecutes white collar crime. It is a fascinating line of work that has allowed me to meet all kinds of people. My work involves participation as a delegate in international securities law, as well as the formulation of policies and legislation that directly affect Canadian investors and those in the investment industry.

At the beginning of a recent session in Madrid, I was particularly delighted when the chairwoman asked me, of her own accord, what steps should be taken to ensure that I could understand the proceedings. In those instances that require me to attend a Commission hearing or court proceedings, the Commissioners and judges have been most gracious in making accommodations so I can understand the entire event and, thus, participate fully and effectively.

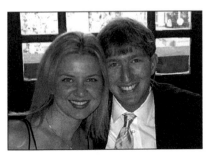

Andrea and I met and fell in love while she was working for the summer at the Alexander Graham Bell Association.

The legal setting can pose challenges. There is great reward in the intellectual stimuli that comes my way; however, it can be difficult for a person with hearing loss to partake in telephone conference calls, or even calls with individuals if they don't speak clearly. The same can be said for meetings, negotiations involving large numbers of people, and so forth. E-mail is a great boon to my practice.

In my spare time I work with various not-for-profit and charitable entities, both locally and internationally, consulting to some and sitting on the board of directors of others. This is highly rewarding, and allows me to bring my legal training to bear in a variety of contexts.

'His Banner Over Me Is Love'

One unexpected and inexpressibly beautiful gift that my hearing loss has brought me is the wonderful woman I love. Andrea and I met under extraordinary circumstances. In January of 2003, I decided to visit Jonathan and Tania and their dear little son Jacob on the day Jacob underwent cochlear implant surgery. Shortly after I got there, Warren arrived, too, and asked if I would be part of a documentary being produced about Jacob's life.

The documentary, titled *Jacob's Journey: The Story of a Nucleus Family*®, was shown at a conference in Baltimore the following summer. Andrea was in the audience and made inquiries at one point about the surgeon. Later, when chatting with Jonathan and Tania, she asked them about their faith and told them about her own. Jonathan and Tania excitedly told her that I shared her Christian faith, whereupon she asked if they would forward her e-mail address to me.

I remember distinctly the hour they told me about her. We were having dinner in their garden and the sky was a glorious blaze of color. I felt an extraordinary peace.

We agreed by e-mail to meet a few weeks later, in Washington, D.C., where she was working for the summer at the Alexander Graham Bell Association for the Deaf and Hard of Hearing. We fell in love. Andrea and I had the most memorable first date — it lasted 5 days! We rented a car and drove 1,600 miles through charming Southern cities such as Cape Hatteras and Asheville, North Carolina, as well as the Blue Ridge Mountains of Virginia, before returning to explore the bustling capital city of Washington. We agree there was no better way to really get to know each other.

Andrea is extraordinary. I quote Proverbs in saying "her worth is far above jewels." Like me, she has a cochlear implant and does amazingly well with it. Andrea and I have been blessed with the ability to hear one another on the phone and carry on endless conversations.

Andrea has just completed her master's degree in teaching and is pursuing studies in deaf education here in Toronto.

We are very fortunate to have been able to travel together. Recently, two good friends were wed in Brazil, which allowed us the opportunity to explore Rio de Janeiro and the stunning Iguaçu Falls that straddle the border of Brazil and Argentina.

Andrea's parents and her lovely sister Marie have recognized the value of lavishing love and wisdom on Andrea. I met Andrea's family for the first time during the Christmas holidays of 2003. Suffice it to say, we bonded quickly and deeply. When I asked her father for permission to court her, he simply said: "All I ask is that you love and cherish my daughter." He then took my hands in his and prayed God's blessings on both of us. Andrea's love for me is wondrously profound. Every day I learn some new and enchanting facet of her character, and I find myself awed and amazed beyond all thought and expression.

Parental Advice

I offer parents the following advice:

- If you instill in your children a sense of wonder and a yearning to explore ideas and places, you give them the world.
- Children should be taught the high value of independence — that is, freedom to think and express oneself creatively, to stand on one's own feet, and to solve problems without the help of others.
- Children should be equipped to educate those with whom they interact — friends, peers, or teachers — to dispel any untruths about hearing loss, and to make others completely at ease in their presence.
- It is far better to be gently and compellingly persuasive than to be aggressively assertive.
- In order to be persuasive, your child must communicate well. In order to communicate well, your child must be able to read well. Embark your child on a lifelong journey of passion for outstanding literature and biographies.

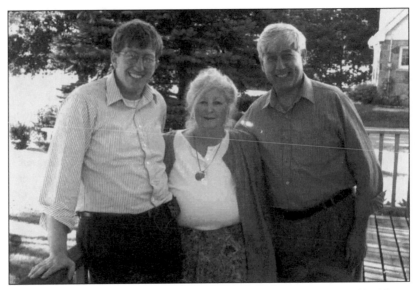

My parents gave me wise and loving counsel about conducting myself with diplomacy, dignity, and grace.

- It is all too easy to "bluff" and "pretend" that you heard something when, in fact, you didn't. Integrity demands that we speak up and clarify when we don't hear.
- Parent groups are wonderful — they bring knowledge, empathy, and friendships.
- Teach your child the value of time, and how to manage it well.
- Always have high and loving expectations. The fact that your expectations are high will stretch your child's mind and talents. The fact that they are loving will give your child the impetus, means, and courage to attain them.

In Conclusion

I often marvel at the good fortune of today's children with hearing loss, with such wide access to state-of-the-art hearing aids and cochlear implants and the prospect that Auditory-Verbal therapy will help them flourish in the hearing world. I recently visited a young girl who had just received a cochlear implant at the Hospital for Sick Children in Toronto. Victoria was only 3 years old at the time. When I saw her sleeping, her beautiful dark hair draped over the pillow, I considered with deep awe the joyous dawn that would soon be hers.

As I look back on the road I have traveled, it is impossible to number all of the phenomenal joys that have blossomed through my hearing loss. I have been introduced to an extraordinary world that is so rich in color and vibrancy, so full of wondrous experiences. I am blessed with incredible friendships and the joy and peace that comes with the assured knowledge that all that I have is because of the endless love, kindness, and untold blessings of Almighty God.

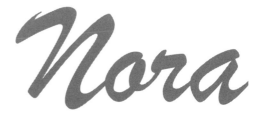

CHAPTER 4

Nora McKellin

THE ABILITY TO HEAR SOUNDS AND CONVERSATION . . . TO LISTEN AND TALK . . . IS taken for granted by so many of those who are not hearing impaired. If you or one of your children is diagnosed with a hearing loss, however, it is not the end of the world. You can get help in listening and speaking, and you can become vitally involved in the hearing world. I don't want to mislead you into thinking it is easy. It takes a lot of work and courage, but it is possible and worth it in the end.

Besides my hearing loss, I have had to learn how to overcome other physical challenges. My life has been difficult, but it has been enlightening and it has made me a stronger and more sensitive person. If I were asked what I would really change about myself, I would have to honestly say that if by some miracle I could be taller, I would choose that. But then again, I am happy with my life. I am only 107 centimeters (approximately $3^1/_2$ feet) tall, and being short is a challenge in a world of full-grown adults. I don't regard my severe-to-profound hearing loss as a major disadvantage, however — at least not anymore! — since I was given an opportunity to participate in Auditory-Verbal therapy at a very early age.

I wear high-powered hearing aids to help me hear, and I am fully engaged in society. I work hard and sometimes get discouraged, but life is very much worth the struggle. I have had a lot of help from some great people along the way, and that's what most of us need, no matter what disappointments or disabilities we must overcome. We can't really go through life all on our own. We need help and encouragement from others. It makes a colossal difference.

Complications from the Start

My twin sister, Meg, and I were born at Women's College Hospital in Toronto on May 15, 1980. We were born prematurely at 35 weeks. My parents expected complications when we were born, but they were not prepared for one child with a form of dwarfism. I weighed 4 pounds-4 ounces; Meg weighed a few ounces less than I did, but my arms and legs were disproportionate and short. She was born healthy and of average height. Later genetic testing determined that even though Meg and I looked quite different, she was indeed my identical twin. The doctors believed I have a rare form of dwarfism called *diastrophic dysplasia.*

With twins to look after, life was very busy for my parents. I also was in and out of hospital with respiratory infections and complications because of a cleft of the soft palate. Until that was repaired when I was 2 years old, feeding me was very complicated.

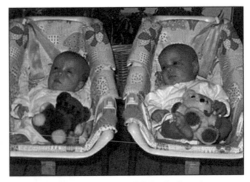

Though Meg (right) and I looked quite different when we were born, she was indeed my identical twin.

Milk used to come out my nose if I was fed too quickly, and I suffered from colic. My mother told me that in those early days of caring for us she was often so tired she was numb!

When I was about 6 months old, the doctors discovered that my upper spinal column was unstable, and it was increasingly difficult for my neck to support my head. At age 2, I was fitted with a back and neck brace. I wore it constantly, except at night when I was in bed, until I was 4.

At 18 months, my parents began to notice that I wasn't responding to words or sounds the way Meg was. In January of 1982, they took me to the ENT clinic at the Hospital for Sick Children in Toronto for a thorough checkup because of persistent ear infections. There, following a brain stem evoked response test, my parents learned the extent of my hearing loss. The test showed a severe-to-profound sensorineural hearing loss of about 80–90 dB in both ears.

My mother said my deafness was more tragic than my other physical problems. For me not to hear a singing bird or music or my parents' voices, and not to be able to tell my parents what I did in school or gossip with my sister, was devastating. The full implications of what a hearing loss meant began to sink in over the next few days and weeks following the diagnosis.

"You keep subtracting from her," my mother said angrily to the doctors, who she felt kept discovering new disabilities every time they took me to the hospital. My parents are very strong and practical people, but they admit they experienced all the same emotions of other families that have children with chronic illnesses or disabilities. They felt anger, sometimes at the doctors and health care givers. They also felt guilt and fear. And, they sometimes felt hopeless. Above all, though, my mother said she felt weary. Looking after Meg and me was a full-time job, and all the visits to the doctor and trips to the therapists and specialists — on top of managing the care-giving required for two young children — was exhausting. My mother didn't work outside the home after we were born, but my father, a professor of anthropology at the University of Toronto, contributed as much as possible when he came home so my mother could have a break.

The intense care-giving was also prolonged because I did not reach the same developmental milestones that Meg did. When Meg was learning to walk, I was still learning to sit up. When Meg was talking and listening, I was still just beginning to babble.

Learning to Listen – and Talk

My parents considered many options for me to acquire speech and language skills. They were aware of the many controversial differences between the educational approaches of Deaf Culture and the hearing world, but they also accepted that following either path depended on family choices and the needs of the individual. After studying all of their options, and after visiting service providers throughout the Toronto area, my parents were convinced that Auditory-Verbal therapy was the right choice for me and our family. They reasoned that I would always be short, and with fused elbows (which limit my mobility) and short fingers, they thought that people might not be able to see me sign and that it might be difficult for me to lipread.

After my diagnosis of hearing loss, I was fitted bilaterally with hearing aids. My mother recounts that I cried when the aids were put on, and I tried to take them off, but little by little I became accustomed to them. When I was 2 years old, my parents and I began to work with Warren Estabrooks, the only Auditory-Verbal therapist at the Learning to Listen Foundation (LTLF) at that time. My mother became my teacher and would go with me to the hospital for our weekly sessions. My parents and I would then practice the lessons at home. Warren systematically guided my mother in helping me to listen, which was essential before I could develop natural speech. I was continuously bathed in sounds and words by my parents. They would comment out loud on everything, narrating all of our daily activities.

The first part of Auditory-Verbal therapy was to try to get me to associate sounds with objects and to make sense out of the sounds that were being amplified by my hearing aids. My mother would seat me at the dining room table in my high chair and place before me a red toy bus, a little plastic cow, and a little yellow-and-blue airplane. She would push it around the table in front of me, saying, "The bus goes bu . . . bu . . . bu." She would pick up the cow and walk it over to me and say, "The cow says moo . . . moo . . . moo." She would fly the airplane toward me and around my head and say, "Listen, the airplane goes ahhhhhhhh." Then she would line up the toys and make the sounds for each, hoping I would pick up the right toy when she made the corresponding sound. Nothing happened for weeks! My mother said she felt down, afraid that this approach was never going to work, but Warren remained confident and encouraging.

Then one day, when my mother was endlessly repeating "bu . . . bu . . . bu," I finally picked up the bus. She took the bus, put it back on the table, and made the sound again . . . and again. I picked it up each time. Then I picked up the cow when she said "moo . . . moo . . . moo," and the airplane when she said "ahhhhhhhh." Matching sounds to objects was a major breakthrough. I progressed through the listening stages to make my own sounds when I saw a familiar object. Soon I began to really listen and to talk — a word at a time. Eventually, I added phrases, then sentences, and then I became so chatty that my parents began to wish I had actually learned to listen a little more and talk a little less.

Beginning School

Another decision my parents made when I was 5 years old was to place Meg and me into a nursery school together for a few days a week. The nursery school accepted children with disabilities and my parents felt that not only would this immerse me in a stimulating and supportive environment, it also would allow me to go to school with my sister.

At the age of 4, I was able to walk on my own, although not for long distances. That was also when I entered kindergarten. It was our local primary school in Toronto, close to our home, and my mother would push me to school in a large, sturdy, upright stroller. My teacher was willing to provide extra assistance and also agreed to work with the FM system. With the help of an itinerant teacher, who came to my classes several times a week, the school staff and my parents felt I would be able to manage in a regular classroom.

During my preschool years, I was still seeing Warren on a weekly basis. I was also trying to get used to using the FM system in school. The receiver had to be worn around my neck or hooked onto my clothing somehow and then the ear jacks were plugged into my hearing aids. The teacher wore a system as well, with a microphone that was supposed to relay her voice directly to my hearing aids, thereby cutting out the background noises that normally would interfere with my ability to hear her. I guess it worked, although wearing the heavy receiver was cumbersome and awkward. On one occasion, a teacher accidentally wore her FM unit to the bathroom!

Not long after kindergarten, my father was offered a job at the University of British Columbia, so we moved out West.

New Home, New Schools

Meg and I were 7 when our family moved to Vancouver, where I was integrated into a first-grade classroom at our neighborhood school. However, my parents decided to place Meg in a nearby French Immersion school. I think this was probably a wise decision since it meant that Meg and I each had the opportunity to live our own lives and make our own circle of friends. I did not have to live in Meg's shadow, nor she in mine. Socially, I got along well with the other students . . . after they got used to me being much shorter than they were. My classmates accepted me and treated me pretty much just like everyone else.

I went to Queen Elizabeth Elementary in Vancouver from first through seventh grades. In my first few years, I wore an FM unit during lessons. The Vancouver School Board also supplied a large rug for the classroom that helped create a positive listening environment. In addition, the school board provided an itinerant teacher, who came to the school 2–3 times a week to give me extra assistance. The itinerant teacher met with the classroom teacher to help her understand my needs, and also met with me outside the classroom to review homework and make sure I understood the vocabulary of certain lessons and projects. We went over new concepts introduced in class, and she assisted me in completing my homework assignments. Writing was sometimes difficult because my hands would tire from holding the pen or pencil, so I needed longer to prepare my homework than other students.

Although most of the classroom teachers were supportive as I moved through the grades, I have to say that a few were not as open-minded as my family had hoped, and my parents sometimes needed to meet personally with school staff and/or a specific teacher. They would ask for meetings with the itinerant teacher and the vice principal (or others) to provide assistance because my regular teachers were either ignoring my needs or making assumptions about what they thought I needed. Mostly, my parents fought to ensure that I had enough support, but not so much that I would lose my independence, or so much to ignore my perspective of how I wanted to be educated.

I had very strong ideas about what worked for me and what did not, and I was not shy about expressing those ideas. My parents respected that and believed I had a right to express my opinions. When I was a bit older, my mother sent me to a "teen independence" camp for disabled teens where I participated in an assertiveness training workshop. "Coals to Newcastle!" my mother said when I got home. "They should have asked *you* to teach that class!"

> When I came back from 'teen independence' camp, my mother said, 'They should have asked *you* to teach that class!'

In school, I wore two hearing aids operated by a small handheld computer that had been specially programmed for me. The computer controlled the volume and response to different background noises. It worked quite well for me, and I generally didn't use other assistive hearing devices. (I didn't use an FM system consistently in either elementary school or high school, and never as a university student. It wasn't very useful because only the teachers would wear the microphone and in the higher grades the classes became more about interacting with other students, none of whom were wearing FM technologies.) I always sat at the front of the class and always faced the person who was talking. I didn't take notes because I couldn't listen and write at the same time; I needed to concentrate carefully on the material being presented. I was always fortunate either to have someone who took notes for me or a teacher who provided written summaries. For assignments, my teachers usually allowed for my spelling problems because it was hard to phonologically sound out certain words. The spell check feature on my computer was wonderful. I used it all the time.

Overall, I would say I was fairly successful in school, but I wasn't a scholar. I wasn't successful at learning other languages. My sister Meg, on the other hand, is bilingual, speaking both French and English. In eighth grade, I took French and managed to get a C+. Unfortunately, in ninth grade, I ended up with an unsympathetic French teacher who had a rigid teaching routine. She did not attempt to alter her methods at all for me. I just couldn't keep up with her rapid oral presentations, nor could I handle the daily dictation exercises that she demanded. I was very unhappy, and my parents and the counselor at school decided it wasn't worth the struggle — that it was better I simply drop the subject.

Forever Friends

I have to be honest in saying that I have encountered people in the schools I attended or in social situations who either pitied me or were ashamed to be seen with me. But, there are always going to be these kinds of people in the world, and you just have to move on. Everyone has encountered "fake" friends, the ones who are very friendly and nice to you at first and then begin to move away, or stop returning your phone calls, or ignore you in school. Nevertheless, I have managed to find some wonderfully close friends in my life. I know we will be friends forever.

My best friend is my sister. She has always been there for me and makes me laugh. She has always been kind to me when I got sick, and even now cheers me up with little surprises when I am feeling blue. She is one of the most dedicated, devoted, and unselfish people I know. When we were kids, she was my unconditional playmate. We always played house, we played dress-up and shared makeup, we played school and library, and made forts. Meg and I are very

My best friend is my sister. She has always been there for me. She is one of the most dedicated, devoted, and unselfish people I know.

similar in some ways, and totally different in others. The obvious difference is that she is taller and doesn't have a hearing loss or any of my physical disabilities. But Meg also doesn't enjoy traveling as much as I do. She is more of a homebody and more studious than I am. I like to see my friends and would rather party than write a paper or read a book. As twins, we are very close. We know each other's moods and have an almost intuitive way of communicating, even without words. But, we are also quite independent and have different sets of friends, different personalities, and different likes and dislikes. I love apple pie and Meg hates it. She loves watermelon and I never eat the stuff. I can stay out until all hours and have been known to party all night. I love sleeping until late in the morning. Meg needs her sleep and has no problem getting up early. I'm very good on the computer but Meg gets easily frustrated with it and constantly calls me to come and fix something.

I can never thank God enough for giving me a twin, and I could not imagine going through life without her. I love her more than life itself. She is my second half and makes me whole.

When I was 9, my sister and I became friends with Meaghan, a new girl in our neighborhood. I remember the day we all met. Her aunt dragged her over to meet us and we were all shy and didn't say much to each other. We all became good friends, however, and the three of us would discuss which house (hers or ours) was having the best meal, and then we would all go there for dinner. Our mothers must have decided to make a little extra each night, in case the three of us were together for dinner. We used to shine flashlights across the street to signal to each other from our bedrooms, and we would play until dark and walk into each other's houses without even knocking. If we were naughty and got grounded, it didn't seem to preclude going to each other's houses. We were known as the "MNM toothless wonders" because somehow we managed to get our teeth pulled at the dentist at the same time. Thirteen years later, we are not just friends, we are more like sisters. We even fight like sisters. Meaghan borrows clothes from Meg, and Meg borrows clothes from her. No one can fit into my clothes so I don't have to worry about that! Or we just hang out in Meaghan's apartment, or she hangs out in ours.

In sixth and seventh grades at Queen Elizabeth Elementary, I met two other wonderful friends: Kali and Karen. We did everything together. Every weekend, we got together at one of our houses, or went to a movie or the mall, or ordered pizza and watched videos. We did things together even when I was at a different high school. We saw each other every weekend and talked every night. This is how I got my own phone line in high school. My father couldn't receive any calls because I was on the phone constantly. If it wasn't someone calling for Meg, it was someone for me. Sometimes my parents wondered out loud, "Why did we ever teach her to talk this much?" I just said, "Well, all that therapy is paying off. Thanks to you guys, I can listen and talk for hours. So be happy!"

I met two other best friends, Tania and Katherine, in 10th grade. In high school, the five of us together were known as "the girls." These friends have greatly influenced the person I have become. They have shown me that they love me for who I am and not for how much or how little I can hear or the way I look. They have taught me that being a friend does not depend on a body. It depends on a mind and a heart. All my friends have looked beyond the surface and searched within. They have eyes to see my soul, not just the physical body. An open heart, an open mind, and an honest soul are the necessary elements for unconditional friendship.

I have also been a nanny for my next door neighbors' children on and off for 11 years. Our family has been close with our neighbors for 17 years. Katy, Laura, and Emma are my three little angels, although I have to admit they are growing up. I have known them since they were born and have looked after them their whole lives. We are all like sisters, too. I love them because they never treated me any differently and they always helped me when I needed them. The whole family shares a special place in my heart.

I have made many friends along my journey, and each has enriched my life in some form. I wish I could name all of them and write how much they mean to me, but then I would go on forever. During my many travels, I have met countless others who share my passion for traveling internationally. They, too, love adventure and the thrill of encountering new places and new cultures. It is important for me to have friends who share my interests.

A Call to Theater

My first high school, which I attended for two years, was such a large school that it was necessary for me to ride my scooter from class to class. I wasn't happy there since I didn't fit in. Everyone was nice to me, but it was hard to make close friends, and it didn't help that two of my best friends from elementary school went to another school.

In high school, I was assigned an itinerant teacher who also was hearing impaired. Even though we shared a common disability, I found it frustrating to work with her because she just wanted to focus on speech lessons. She never set a regular time to see me, often arriving right when I was in the middle of something important. And, since she never wanted to come into the classroom with me, I had to get up and go to another classroom. I felt I didn't need to be drilled on speaking techniques; I needed less therapy and more practical support — someone who was prepared to go over class notes with me and make sure I had understood the instructions correctly.

Even before I met her, I discovered that this itinerant teacher had called the school to change my entire timetable to better accommodate her schedule rather than mine. This timetable switch conflicted with the schedule I had developed with my disability resources teacher, which was based on ensuring that I had a solid safety route and sufficient time for me to get from class to class in a three-story building of more than 2,000 students. My parents, my disability resources teacher, and the school counselor finally decided that I would work only with my disability resources teacher and would no longer need the assistance of the itinerant teacher.

Despite the supportive teachers and counselors, my parents realized at the end of ninth grade that I was not at all happy at that school. They lobbied successfully with the Vancouver School Board to allow me to transfer to another school just outside the catchment area for where we lived. University Hill (U Hill) was a smaller school, but with two of my best friends there already, it was easier to make new friends and get involved in school life. One of my best friends encouraged me to join the school theater company. Over the next three years, I was intensely involved in theater as the promotions manager, house manager, assistant director, and director. I also worked in stage management and costume and set design.

> The theater really helped bring out the hidden person inside me. Working in theater taught me independence and raised my self-esteem.

When I worked as a stagecraft manager, two of my duties were to run the show and call the show. That meant operating the lights and sound according to each scene. To accommodate my hearing loss, a classmate sat next to me in the technical booth (rather than staying backstage) so I could see the stage manager giving me lighting or sound cues to run the show. Sometimes I wore headphones and watched a video camera so I could see and hear the stage manager signaling backstage and giving cues for the show. I used these techniques because I didn't want to let down the rest of the team or mess up the show because I had missed hearing one of the cues.

I also completed a provincially acknowledged Career Preparation Program in Performance Arts and Productions by working at least 100 hours in local theaters. In this program, I worked in a community theater group for two years, directed a segment on the television program "Stargate SG-1," and also worked at the Vancouver Opera. University Hill named me Student of the Term two years in a row, and in 12th grade I was nominated as Drama Leadership Student of the Year. I also received a community service medal and an honor roll certificate my final year.

It was the theater that really helped bring out the hidden person inside me. Working in theater taught me independence, helped me develop leadership skills, taught me how to take initiative, and raised my self-esteem and confidence. I believe that everyone should take on some sort of leadership role early in life because it is such good preparation for the real world challenges of university and an eventual career.

In June of 1999, I graduated from University Hill with several awards: the Ceramics 12 Scholarship, the Drama Leadership Scholarship, and an Arbutus Rotary Scholarship of $500. The Rotary Scholarship is based on good marks and community service. When the awards were announced, I happened to be sitting in the back row and couldn't hear when my name was called. Consequently, I never really heard the nice things that were said about me. One of my friends kept kicking me to let me know that my name had been called, and then I had to run backstage the long way round to get out in front again. It was quite an exciting time; my parents and my sister, my grandmother from Chicago, my disability resources teacher, and Meaghan were all in the audience clapping like mad. My mother was crying.

A Passion for Traveling

My hobbies include watching movies, hanging out with friends, ceramics, reading, sewing, knitting, and writing poetry. However, I am passionate about traveling. I have traveled in Canada, the United States, Australia, and Europe. In the United States, the trips have been mainly to visit my parents' family and friends I met on a trip to Australia. All my aunts, uncles, cousins, and grandparents live in the United States, some in the Boston area, some outside of Chicago, and others near Harrisburg, Pennsylvania. I miss my extended family because I don't see them very often, so I love it when I can visit them.

In 1998, I went on a cultural exchange trip to Australia. I stayed with an Australian family for two weeks and spent another two weeks on a bus tour with fellow students from North America and France. I made some wonderful friends on my visit, traveling from the Great Barrier Reef to Sydney, and remain in touch with many of them today. In 2000, in fact, I traveled to western Europe with a girl from Canada and two from the United States whom I had met in Australia. Our male friends from France who were in the exchange program invited us to visit them whenever the opportunity arose, so we did. Some of our friends lived on the west coast of France and another had a fabulous beach house on the French Riviera! Four of us traveled throughout France and Switzerland, and then my friend, Tarah, and I traveled to Italy and Germany. After that, we met my parents and Meg in Paris and I traveled with them throughout England.

It's a small world; I ran into so many people in Europe that I knew from Vancouver. When my friend Jodie and I arrived at the airport in Paris, we weren't quite sure how to get into the city, so I went up to two young men and asked for directions. One of them looked down at me and said, "Nora, is that you? What are you doing here?" Jodie said, "How do you know someone already and we're only five minutes off the plane?" They were two boys I knew from high school! Another time, at a hostel, I was sitting at the computer in the lobby when someone came up behind me and gave me a hug. I turned around to discover it was one of my friends from University Hill who was there picking up some friends!

Travel Liberates

Travel liberates the physical body.
People's minds need to widen to perceptions, to solutions, to
    adaptations.
It is in the art of dealing with unexpected situations.
It is a mental, a physical and a spiritual game.
People who are seen as different have mastered the artistry of
    embracing challenges,
Have mastered the artistry of dominating circumstances,
Have mastered to deal with the stares and invisibility,
And defining and demanding a standard of respect.
To be Human.
Travel liberates
A sense of purpose, a sense of importance,
A sense of destination, a sense of accomplishment,
A sense of fulfillment, a sense of higher knowledge.
The soul searches for self empowerment and utmost
    independence.
Travel liberates the mind to travel with other minds.
Travel forces one to look deeper into one's surroundings not
    just exterior bodies.
Travel coerces one to inspect intensely,
To show people that physical limitation does not mean
    confinement, nor negativism,
Nor the inability to do nothing.
One's own boundaries of self-limitations and exploration.
It's a cycle of adventure, a love affair that doesn't have to end.

(N. McKellin)

When I first arrived in Paris, I forgot to call my parents to let them know that I had arrived safely. My mother, of course, was worried. After two days, she called the Three Ducks Hostel where I was supposed to be staying and asked for Eleanor McKellin. The receptionist said, "No, there is no one here by that name." Then my mother asked, "Well, is there someone named Nora there? "Oh, Nora?!" the receptionist replied. "Oh yes, there is a Nora here — very petite, very lively, very healthy, very happy." "OK," my mother said, relieved. "Just tell her that her mother's glad she's still alive."

Giving Something Back

In April of 2002, Warren invited me to speak at the VOICE for Hearing Impaired Children (VOICE) conference in Kitchener, Ontario, near Toronto. It was a great experience to come back to my birthplace and to the place where I had first learned to listen and talk. I had not been to the Toronto area since 1987. I was so nervous because I wanted to do the best I could for Warren and was touched and grateful that he had asked me to do the speech. In fact, I really don't think I could ever turn down anything he asked me to do. He is, after all, very persuasive.

I also felt very happy to know that now I could give something back to others after all the help I have been given. It was an honor to have an opportunity to share my story with others, and to be able to tell parents of children who are deaf that listening and talking is not an impossible dream for their children. With dedication and perseverance, anything is possible!

A month later, I was a youth leadership participant at the Canadian

Hard of Hearing Association conference in Ottawa, attending workshops designed to help students build leadership skills. This was another amazing experience! I was surrounded by people who could not talk, who signed or who did a bit of both, or just talked and listened like me. I have never known many people who were deaf or hard of hearing. Because I went to a neighborhood school and none of my classmates were deaf, this experience was both enlightening and challenging since I had to figure out different modes of communication.

In August of 2003, my father and I where asked to be guest lecturers for the Little People of BC conference, and I had to prepare my speech less than 12 hours after my sister's wedding. This was another eye-opening experience since it was the first time I had really been around other short people. I still keep in touch with friends I made at that conference.

Gaining a Different Perspective

In 1999, I enrolled at the University of British Columbia, although I almost didn't get in because I missed that year's competitive grade point cutoff for the Faculty of Arts by 1%. I had a 75% and the school was admitting those with 76% and above. On my behalf, many of my high school teachers wrote supportive letters to the university, and after the associate dean of arts reviewed my file, I was admitted under the broader-based admissions policy. UBC was my first choice of universities because my sister Meg was already a student there, as were some of my friends from high school.

I received a number of support services from UBC's Disability Resource Centre. Because of my physical limitations, I rearranged some of my classes to more accessible classroom locations. I had the use of a computer on loan, I received extra time for exams, and I received assistance from notetakers, a service paid for by the university. I also was able to use some of my friends as notetakers, along with Meg, who took a few classes with me. UBC is the first school Meg and I have attended together since we were in play school.

I majored in sociology, and followed an interest in how social systems, health care, education, tourism, and the media are interrelated. My experiences gave me a different perspective, which helped me in sociology. I saw things that other people took for granted. I shared my experiences and perspective with medical students in the UBC Faculty of Medicine as an interviewee on disability issues.

Critical Challenges

Most of my challenges are physical. I was born short-limbed, with a curved spine, and when I was young I wore a neck- and back-brace for four years. I do not have elbow joints, and I had a cleft palate that was corrected with plastic surgery when I was 2 years old. I have had many ear infections and respiratory complications. I have had pneumonia five times already, and once almost died from a serious case of bronchitis. Although I have had more than nine surgeries to date, my back operation and my ear surgery were the most critical.

I have both scoliosis and kyphosis of the spine. In December of 1990, I underwent critical reconstructive spinal surgery because the curve of my spine increased unexpectedly. I had two major operations, but it was done in four parts (in other words, it was four back operations). I underwent the first part of the operation on December 3, and was in the intensive care unit for more than a week because of a collapsed lung and because I had a bad reaction when the doctors gave me too much morphine. The second part of the operation was delayed for several weeks because of further complications.

I was released from the hospital on December 23, just in time for Christmas, and arrived home in an ambulance. I spent nine months lying flat on my back and was sandbagged into place to keep my spine from moving. During the night, I had to be turned over every four hours. My parents alternated nights sleeping next to me and turning me over. Subsequently, I had to wear a trunk and head brace for two years. It wasn't until August that I was finally allowed to begin walking again.

During my recuperation, I was visited at home by an itinerant teacher, who worked on lessons with me, gave me homework, and then checked it the following week. With this assistance, I was able to return to school without missing a grade. I must admit, however, that the two major back surgeries were the hardest things I have endured.

As I said above, I also have had many ear infections over the years. During an ear examination in August of 2002, my ENT doctor noticed a shadow behind my eardrum. He suspected a buildup of dead skin over the bones of my middle ear and ordered a CT scan. The scan showed that I had a cholesteatoma, a noncancerous growth. I had surgery to remove it. Since I am small and have narrow airways, the surgery was a little more complicated than it is for other people. The worst part of the surgery, however, was the recovery time of eight weeks. I could not wear my hearing aid in that ear for two months. That was very difficult because the tumor was on my better ear.

Not being able to hear as well was a unique experience, but it was also very trying. It is much easier to cope with something that you never had. I went from hearing a lot to hearing almost nothing. I was struggling with the notion of not being able to hear and it changed who I was during that time.

Another change occurred during this period. I had to depend on a new form of communication (closed captioning) while taking two courses at UBC, so I experienced first hand both the hardships and the positive aspects of not being able to hear. I now have real-life experience as both a hearing person and a deaf person. Being hearing impaired presents a world that is neither totally hearing nor totally deaf. It is a world that bridges the two. I misplace my hearing aids every once in a while, and I always have to get new molds. Sometimes the hearing aids just stop working. My family gets frustrated with me at these moments when they can't get my attention or make themselves understood.

There are a number of advantages to not being able to hear, however. For instance, I can turn off my hearing aids any time and anywhere, which allows me to enter a world of calming silence. With my aids off, I always get a soundless

> I went from hearing a lot to hearing almost nothing. I was struggling with the notion of not being able to hear and it changed who I was.

sleep, and I can study anywhere no matter how noisy it is or use closed captioning to watch TV silently while someone, such as my sister, is asleep in the same room. I have also learned to play "Jingle Bells" with the feedback from my hearing aids, a skill that always goes over well at parties. And, I always win lipreading competitions.

I use two devices on a regular basis because of my hearing loss: a doorbell that flashes and plays a song (which means I can hear it even without my hearing aids) and a very loud alarm clock that flashes lights in my face to wake me up.

Once in high school, I had a sleepover with some friends and we were watching a scary movie. Meg came home with a couple of her friends and tried to frighten us by scratching on the window, which got us all screaming. Meg's friends also decided to sleep over that night, so I was able to get my sweet revenge! Two of her friends were planning to sleep in the upstairs room next to mine. While they were downstairs, I sneaked up the stairs and set my alarm clock for 4 a.m., turning up the volume to its loudest intensity. At the selected hour, the clock emitted its deafening siren and flashed its lights everywhere. At first, Meg's friends thought it was a fire alarm or the police. When they discovered it wasn't, they began running around the room pulling plugs from every socket trying to stop the noise. The next morning, I asked them innocently, "Did you boys have a good sleep last night?"

Return to Australia

In January of 2003, I began a three-month UBC student exchange program to the University of Queensland in Brisbane, Australia. I planned to study the sociology of tourism, globalization and technology in addition to Australian popular culture. School didn't start until March so before going to our respective exchange schools, I traveled around New Zealand for two weeks with my friend, Scott, a fellow student from UBC. In New Zealand, we took the Kiwi Experience Bus Tour and visited Auckland, Whitianga, Taupo, Rotorua, and Wellington. My favorite adventure was in Tashtego Falls near Rotorua. We went for a two-hour hike between two volcanoes. We walked a path that took us in and out of forests and to a stream that led to the falls. I had some difficulty negotiating some of the stairs — some were as high as my shoulders! Thank goodness for Scott's helping hand. The view was spectacular and, more important, we were the only people on the tour to actually hike up the falls! I was amazed that I could push beyond my physical limitations and see the world from a different perspective.

Landing back in Australia, we met up with my friend Kali and the three of us went traveling for another four weeks. That proved to be more of an adventure than we had anticipated. After a long bus ride from Melbourne to Adelaide, we decided to rent a car to journey to Sydney. The car was not in the best shape, and after we left Melbourne its condition went downhill quickly. We nicknamed her "Old Bessie" since she looked rather like a cream-colored cow. Old Bessie kept getting overheated, and we had to stop

> I have also learned to play 'Jingle Bells' with the feedback from my hearing aids, a skill that always goes over well at parties.

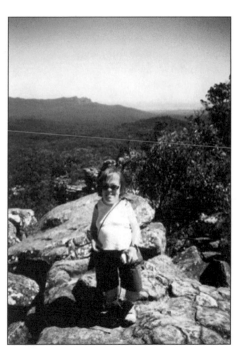

Stopping to enjoy the view while hiking in the Grampian Mountains in Victoria.

frequently to cool her off. We filled her with many bottles of coolant and an endless amount of gas!

When we began climbing the Snowy Mountains, Old Bessie joined the roadkill by dying on the steep highway. There wasn't much traffic in the area, and after 30 minutes of trying to flag down help, a trucker hauling 400 live sheep finally stopped! We hitched a ride with the sheep, but the trucker was headed in the opposite direction so he called his brother to come and get us. His brother picked us up and returned us to our car, but we had to wait several hours for the tow truck in the pitch-black night with the sounds of animals echoing around us. The tow truck finally arrived and took us to the next town, Adaminaby (also known as the home of the world's largest trout). The three of us spent the entire next day in the garage waiting for a verdict on the car. The mechanic finally told us that Old Bessie wouldn't be going anywhere anymore. The only way out of town, therefore, was to hitch a ride on the Adaminaby school bus — one bus served the whole Snowy Mountains district! — to Cooma. We then took a bus to Canberra and then Sydney.

So, how many people can say that they have been stranded in the middle of the Snowy Mountains and rescued by 400 sheep? Only us three.

In our month of traveling, we visited Sydney, Melbourne, Adelaide, the Yaldarra Valley, the Barossa Valley, the Grampian Mountains, and the Great Ocean Road, as well as many smaller towns such as Wagga Wagga. After finally arriving in Sydney, we stayed with my friend Jodie for a week, then all went our separate ways: Kali back to Vancouver, Scott to study in Melbourne, and me to do the same in Brisbane. It was quite lonely in the beginning, but I had a blast in the end and found it very hard to leave all the great friends I met over there. It helped especially when a friend from Ottawa came and lived with me for two months in my small bachelorette suite.

The family that had served as my hosts on my first trip to Australia in 1998 made sure I got settled again this time, particularly when they helped me buy the big bulky stuff that I needed for the next few months. I signed up to be part of the Chocolate Society Club, which is where I met Brigit and Jema. It was my dream club! We spent all our time watching movies and eating chocolate! I hung out with Brigit and Jema most of the time, and even went dancing with them every weekend. I also became friends with other residents in my apartment building, especially my neighbor, Sarah.

Scott came to visit at the semester break and we traveled to Fraser Island and Byron Bay. Then Tania arrived from Vancouver for three weeks to help celebrate my birthday. It was a very special way to celebrate with familiar faces and newly made friends.

Perth was my last major adventure with Tania and Scott. We rented a four-berth Winnebago to visit Fremantel, Augusta, and Margaret River (before visiting Rottenest Island on my own). Unfortunately, I came down with pneumonia. Scott and Tania put up with my coughing, and were very patient and took good care of me. I felt bad that I put a damper on the trip, but they never once got upset or angry. Then they got sick and had to cancel their plans to go diving up the coast at Exmouth. They have never held it against me, and I will always remember their kindness.

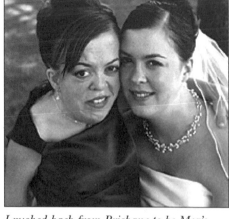

I rushed back from Brisbane to be Meg's maid of honor. I wouldn't have missed her wedding for the world!

During our Winnebago adventure, we went hiking through limestone caves, went whale watching on an incredibly terrifying stormy day, and visited the Valley of the Giants Walk. In retrospect, it was like an out-of-body experience. I finally flew back to Brisbane, packed my bags, bid a difficult goodbye to my new friends, and headed home to Canada — all in the same week.

I rushed home from Australia to see my sister, Meg, get married. Even though I didn't want to leave Brisbane, I wouldn't have missed her wedding for the world. I was Meg's maid of honor, and it was the most beautiful wedding. I have known Andrew, Meg's husband, since fourth grade. I remember that he was the only person in my class who visited me in the hospital after my back surgery. He also brought me cupcakes on Valentine's Day.

I am so happy they have found one another; and that they are so devoted to each other. Meg has someone else in her life who loves her as much as I do.

Life Today

I completed my undergraduate degree in sociology in July 2004, and then finished the rest of my arts degree requirements in September. I was completely done with my studies in December, but had to wait until May 2005 to graduate officially since UBC has only two convocations a year.

As I write this, I have begun looking into graduate school. I wasn't sure what I would be doing. I either want to work on a master's degree in critical disability studies or social policy concerning people with disabilities, or pursue a master's in social work. I am interested in how education and social government policy have shaped the lives of people with disabilities.

Eventually, I would like to get a degree in travel management. Traveling, I believe, helps open one's eyes to the whole world. I want to develop my own business or become a disability consultant specializing in travel for people of short stature. There is a preconceived notion that disability travel only pertains to people in wheelchairs, but help is not available for many types of disabilities. I want to use my training in sociology to assist other students with disabilities pursue their interests and figure out ways to fund their travel dreams. There are so many restrictions and health issues when one leaves the country. There is a great need for public awareness.

No words can truly express my gratitude to my mother, my father, and my sister. They have all made sacrifices for me. My mother dedicated herself to helping me through Auditory-Verbal therapy and also resigned from her job to care for me during the long recovery period following my back surgery. My father has taken me to many, many doctors' appointments and tests. Meg has been my unconditional best friend through all the hard times. I realize that it has not been easy for her to have a sister with a disability, and she has sometimes struggled for the attention that I was getting. I am blessed to have such an extraordinary, devoted family.

My family's support and faith in me have made me who I am today. When things got tough, my mother always said, "Bite the bullet and just keep on." My parents always told me just because I was short and hearing impaired, it should never stop me from following my dreams. They said I could be anything I wanted to be if I got a good education and worked hard.

I am enormously grateful to my friends and therapists, but I am alive and doing well today because of God . . . because of many miracles of grace, both large and small. I believe I could not have overcome so many obstacles or learned to understand myself if I did not have God looking out for me.

Without the devotion of Warren early in my life — his love of teaching and his special friendship — I would not have learned how to listen and talk. Learning how to listen and talk empowered me to pursue my dreams and express who I am.

> Treat your child who is deaf just like other kids. They may be different, but they have the same feelings, thoughts, and spiritual needs.

A Message for Parents

Hardships can bring out the worst in people, but they can also bring out the best. If any of you have been through the worst and come out of it a better person, you know it's worth it in the end. In my experience, people who do not go through hard times, do not value life the same way. Those of us who have had to struggle for our lives really appreciate all its joys as well as its sorrows.

My advice to parents is to treat your child who is deaf just like other kids. They may be different, but they have the same feelings, thoughts, and spiritual needs that all children do. They have minds; they have souls. Encourage them to dream and teach them to dream. It will be hard to let go when they can stand on their own and they start doing their own thing! But, just remember that without your dedication and love, they would be somewhere else. Your child will stumble! So let them stumble, and let them grow to become independent. The hardest thing for a parent is the letting go. Embrace the process and the outcome will be life rewarding.

I conclude with the following poem:

I am a human who is a wonder and who wonders.
I am a human who has strived with faith and redefined the odds.
I am a human who longs to revolutionize society's views,
Who is determined to execute her best to achieve beyond natural boundaries,
redefining limitations.
I am a human who is trapped in a corpse unsuitable to personality, yet whose
body defines character.
I am a human who is free to listen and hear sounds.
I am a human with a lucidity of purpose and power.
I am a human who sees within, a sense of difference from others.
I am a human who has an ambition to alter the illusions of humanity.

CHAPTER 5

Richard

Richard William Orello Farr

"From the moment of birth, the hearing impaired infant begins a life-long quest for satisfying, meaningful relationships with other human beings. . . . Indeed, the extent to which children become successful, participating members of their culture is in direct proportion to the degree to which they are accepted by their families, their peers, their schools, their churches, their communities and to the degree that they are capable of accepting themselves as worthy persons."

IN NOVEMBER OF 1973, THOSE PROFOUND WORDS WERE PUBLISHED BY THE ALEXANDER Graham Bell Association for the Deaf in the abstract, "Here I Am World: Let Me In." For my mother, those words would hold special meaning. In fact, they defined her mission in raising me.

A Rare Survivor

It wasn't supposed to happen like this. In September of 1967, my mother was rushed to Wellesley Hospital in Toronto. Seven months pregnant, she had just returned from a wonderful family holiday at Expo '67 in Montreal, but now she had a high fever and needed immediate attention. At the hospital, she was treated and seemed to be recovering when, a few days later, she went into labor and gave birth to me. I was born at 28 weeks gestation, weighing 2 pounds-9 ounces. Since I was not expected to make it through the night, I was quickly baptized.

Several hours after birth, I was transferred by taxi to the nearby Hospital for Sick Children, since Wellesley Hospital didn't have the facilities to adequately care for such a premature baby. In the 1960s, medical technology was much different than it is today and premature babies usually didn't survive.

My physical appearance at birth was normal, although, of course, I was quite small. I was prone to apnea spells, however, and would frequently stop breathing. When this happened, the nurses would race down the hall and pull a string attached to my ankle to remind me to breathe — an unusual alarm system, but one that worked. The nurses fondly nicknamed me "Richard the Lion Hearted" because of my perseverance. After three months in intensive care, my condition finally stabilized and I was moved into the nursery (though it was against my mother's wishes). At one point in the nursery, my heart stopped, and since I was no longer being monitored as strictly, it took a while before someone noticed and resuscitated me. I spent 10 days in the nursery before I was finally released from the hospital, making it home in time for my first Christmas. By New Year's Day, I weighed 5 pounds. For the next nine months, until I turned 1, I was kept on a strict diet where I was breast fed every three hours.

When I came home from the hospital, my parents were very wary of any potential physical or cognitive problems I might have. Since I had been born three months premature, I was cognitively three months behind in my development. Any suspicions my parents had about my hearing or other possible ailments may have been excused by my delayed development.

Although I apparently acted like a normal baby — very much like my brother, who was two-and-a-half years my senior — my parents had a gut feeling that something wasn't quite right. If I couldn't see my parents, for instance, I wouldn't stop crying until they touched my shoulder, even if they were calling my name. That first summer, my mother set up a playpen on the front lawn (which you could do in those days) and put me in it so I could watch people and cars go by while she cooked in the kitchen. Once when my mother heard a dog barking, she went outside to find it at the edge of the playpen barking incessantly at my back while I happily played with my toys. I didn't even know the dog was there, and it was at that moment that my mother knew this was a serious issue that couldn't be ignored.

Choosing the Oral Approach

My parents were devastated when they realized something was wrong, but my mother quickly began working on finding ways to help me. At first, I underwent rudimentary hearing tests that consisted of a doctor shaking a bell and clapping beside my ear before proclaiming, "Yes, he is deaf." In the 1960s, technology that could accurately measure hearing was extremely rare, so we did not know the extent of my hearing loss for some time. However, a neighbor of ours who taught oral therapy to children at the Toronto School for the Deaf gave us guidance on available options that might help. Traditionally, there were two communication methods for children who are deaf: the Total Communication (TC) method and the oral communication (OC) method. Neither method had a reputation for reliability, however. With the OC method, children could rarely speak intelligibly enough to be understood by individuals with normal hearing, and with the TC method, most "hearing" people could not understand sign language.

At most boarding schools that taught oral communication, students were not allowed to sign to each other and would be punished if they were caught doing so. Thus, the students could't understand each other verbally and the only way they could communicate was to make up their own sign language. That meant that after they finished the OC program they would either be isolated from the "hearing" community because no one could understand them or they would integrate into the "deaf" community where no one could understand them either since they didn't have a common sign language. The development of the hearing aid allowed the oral student to receive stimulus from sound by training his or her residual hearing. Unfortunately, this type of training didn't become a regular part of the OC program for some time, even though oral students in the 1960s wore hearing aids. My mother didn't want me to go away to a boarding school and we were also moving to Winnipeg at that time, so instead I was enrolled in the correspondence course from the John Tracy Clinic in Los Angeles.

The actor Spencer Tracy, whose son was deaf, founded the John Tracy Clinic. His wife wanted to develop a program where she could reach out and teach oral communication to parents of children who were deaf. In June of 1964, the clinic conducted a survey of schools for the deaf in the United States in order to determine the level of education these children were achieving. The survey found that most students ages 16 and older graduated with about a fifth-grade level of education. In comparison, a 16-year-old with normal hearing typically would have an 11th-grade education. The survey clearly showed how little education students who were deaf were receiving at these schools. Officials at the clinic wanted to change that.

Initially, the John Tracy Clinic taught oral education through correspondence, which was perfect for my mother and for other parents living far away from California. At that time, we had moved to Winnipeg, a city without any teachers of the deaf. The clinic provided my family with the resources needed to get started. My mother would receive a lesson book every month and would report on my progress. Teachers at the clinic would then write back to my mother with any advice and guidance, a process that went on for some time. The motto behind the lessons was "TALK, TALK, TALK." I also learned how to lipread. No effort was made to emphasize the use of hearing aids or training so individuals could take advantage of their residual hearing.

> My mother wrote that when I was 19 months old I was 'an exceptionally happy and even-tempered baby and had an incredible amount of patience.'

I received my first hearing aids when I was 16 months old. They were two huge boxes that ran on AA batteries, and my mother had to make a "bra" for me so I could wear them on my chest. Within two weeks, I was saying "uhp-uhp" to get attention, which was a remarkable achievement. Then, at 19 months, I reached another milestone when I started to walk, and it was about this time that my mother wrote the following to officials at the clinic: "[Richard] was an exceptionally happy and even-tempered baby and had an incredible amount of patience."

My mother adopted many of the exercises suggested by experts at the John Tracy Clinic, including the one in which a balloon was held to my head so I could feel the sound vibrations when my mother spoke. My mother also helped me learn to lipread by getting me to look at her face before she spoke. Slowly, I developed sounds, words, language, and lipreading skills. By the summer of 1970, when I was 33 months old, I had developed a vocabulary of 21 words. (In contrast, my hearing daughter — who, as I write this, is 31 months — can say up to 8 words in a sentence and has a vocabulary in the hundreds.) When I attended the John Tracy Clinic with my mother that summer, staff members there said they were surprised I had such an extensive vocabulary.

Attending the clinic was beneficial for my mother and me. She met some amazing and inspirational people who helped her focus on the difficult task of raising me. She learned two very important statements: "Take the *e* out of emotion" (i.e., when you have a problem, do something about it); and "Spend at least 20 minutes with each immediate family member every day."

I remember many occasions on which I caused my parents grief because of my inability to hear. Once, I saw my father working in the backyard and tapped on the window to get his attention. Since I couldn't hear how hard to tap, I actually knocked so hard that I broke the glass. I remember several trips with my father to the hardware store to replace the glass. My mother remembered another occasion when she was driving down the highway and heard a banging noise. Looking into the backseat, she realized that I had found a hammer and was banging on the window. I'm also told that I constantly made an extremely annoying screeching noise. Fortunately, that ceased before I was 3 years old.

I attended my first nursery school in Winnipeg when I was 28 months old. My mother wrote the following in a letter to the John Tracy Clinic:

> *"I really felt he might play strange or go wildly around the room not accomplishing anything, but no, to him it's just a wonderful big party."*

In April of 1971, after my family had moved back to Toronto, I started working with my first real teacher at the Hospital for Sick Children: Louise Crawford. I had a vocabulary of more than 150 words, which was exceptional for my age, especially for someone with profound hearing loss. (Of course, a similarly aged child with normal hearing would have a vocabulary of more than 2,000 words.) Miss Crawford was my introduction to Auditory-Verbal therapy. My mother said the other day that she wished I had started my therapy at 16 months rather than 3½ years. That, she believes, would have made a difference in the clarity of my present-day speech.

I was never held back growing up. My parents did their best to build my confidence even when other parents watched in discomfort seeing me do things ahead of my years. My mother believed in the adage "Better a broken bone than a broken spirit," so she always made sure I did the same things as my brother when he was my age. My parents wanted me treated as a child with normal hearing and not to be overly protected because of my disability. They were never upset even when I went swimming or sailing while wearing my expensive hearing aids. Instead, they would pull out the hair dryer and dry them if I returned dripping wet.

My parents always made everything seem like an adventure. They believed that I had to feel good about myself since physically there was nothing wrong

> My parents did their best to build my confidence even when other parents watched in discomfort seeing me do things ahead of my years.

with me other than my hearing loss. They knew I needed self-confidence to cope with the stress of dealing with deafness in everyday life. Because of their hard work and support, I never doubted my ability to face new challenges even when I knew it might be beyond my current abilities.

One of my all-time favorite pastimes is reading, which I enjoy more than anything else. I have every reason to believe that reading was instrumental in developing my language skills and awareness of the world. Reading gave me "clues" on human behavior, such as how to interact with people and the importance of developing social skills. It also helped develop my imagination. Most children could learn language naturally, but a child like me could not and had to make up the difference through reading. Reading came naturally to me — I didn't require any encouragement from my parents. To this day, I read the paper and check the news on the Internet throughout the day, but nothing beats a good novel.

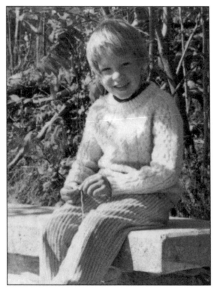

Here I am in 1972. My mother believed in the adage "Better a broken bone than a broken spirit." She made sure I did the same things as my brother when he was my age.

Best of Friends

I met my best friend in fourth grade. When school started, the teacher was wondering where to seat me, and since it seemed no one wanted to sit beside me, she gave me a desk beside Steve — the loudest kid in the class. Naturally he was not initially pleased with the teacher's decision, but he soon realized that I was a great person and we got along really well from that point. Two weeks later, I invited him to my parents' cottage at Sturgeon Lake and we had a wonderful time. Steve soon became one of the few people in the school who could understand me. Often when I answered a question, the teacher would ask Steve to repeat what I had said, and if Steve knew I had given the wrong answer, he would say the correct one. (No wonder I got good marks!) We have been best friends ever since.

My brother Jamey tells me that some individuals occasionally teased him by calling him "Haaayymeeee," mimicking the way I said his name. Jamey didn't take kindly to that and would sometimes respond to these taunts physically, and they never teased him after that. Once people got to know me, however, they discovered that I was just like everyone else. I don't remember being bullied or teased. I may have been teased, of course, but I didn't hear it. Ironically, the person who teased me the most was Steve. One day, I got tired of his teasing and kneed him in the stomach. He never teased me again.

Steve was a great guy and could see that I was naive in many ways. He took it upon himself to develop my understanding of the world — to make me "street smart."

Expanding My Horizons

In the summer of 1974, I joined the local sailing club near my parents' cottage. The following summer, I met my first girlfriend at that club and we spent the whole summer together. I sailed every day of every summer for the next 10 years, finding my place as an equal in a wonderful group of comrades, all of whom had normal hearing. We remain a very close group of friends today.

I take great pride in the fact I received my sailing certificates at the same rate as my "hearing" friends. I was also on my club's racing team for three summers, competing throughout Ontario.

When I finished high school in 1986, I became a sailing instructor and worked during the summer at the club. I enjoyed many great experiences that year, especially one memorable regatta in Kingston, Ontario, where I was able to stay at a family's home for the weekend. The family was very nice and even set up their stereo system with headphones so I could listen to music without wearing my hearing aids. They couldn't believe how loud they needed to turn it up. Apparently they could hear the music through the earphones from the other side of the house. I was particularly fond of Billy Joel's music, so much that my friend Kate took time to write out the lyrics for me.

Another moment of growth for me came in 1979 when the Canadian Hearing Society approached my mother to ask whether I would be interested in acting in *The Miracle Worker* at Toronto's Young Peoples Theatre. The cast was made up mostly of children who were blind or deaf. I jumped at the chance and had a great time. It was like living a dream. Between rehearsals, everybody just played together. I also didn't have to go to school and I got paid. Fortunately, despite missing two months of school, I was able to stay on top of my schoolwork.

A Joyful Time

Of all my time in school, seventh and eighth grades were my favorites. My best friend, Steve, also attended the Montcrest School; however, he started there in the spring and was able to "break the ice" with my class before I arrived in the fall.

I have many good memories of those two years. I remember one time in music class when the teacher asked the students to bring a recorder to school so we could learn how to play it. The next day, I showed up with a tape recorder. I enjoyed learning how to play the recorder and thought I did well keeping in time with everyone else. Steve tells me I wasn't very good, so I guess maybe people were just tolerating me.

I also enjoyed playing hockey, but I couldn't hear when the others would call out "Pass the puck" or "Watch out." Therefore, I would simply skate to the best of my ability and pass the puck when I could. We also played Red Rover. In this game, two teams stand facing each other in a line with their arms interlinked. Someone calls out "Red Rover, Red Rover" and says the name of a person on the other team. That person must leave his line and run across the playground trying to break through the other line. If he breaks through, he returns to his own side and takes someone from the other team with him; if not, he must stay with the other team. The game goes on until one team has all the players on its side.

I was never good at this game since I couldn't hear the other team call my name. Because of that, they allowed for a "pause" period in which the person beside me would tell me whether it was my turn to cross. I didn't get called much, but the important thing was that I was involved.

Self-Awareness

I don't think I became aware of other people's perception of my disability until the fall of 1981 when I entered ninth grade at the Crescent School in Toronto. That was when I first started feeling self-conscious. Upon reflection, I think it was the combination of a number of things: starting a new school, not knowing anyone at the school, being a teenager, and developing an increased awareness of the world.

The first week of high school was not an easy transition for me. Two days after school started, I came down with a bad case of poison ivy. I had a rash from head to toe and was on the verge of being hospitalized. As a result, I missed two weeks of school and eventually went back on crutches because the scabs from the poison ivy hurt my legs. (Until I healed, I often had to leave school early because of the discomfort.) Nevertheless, my teachers were impressed with my attitude and admired my perseverance.

In ninth grade, my studies weren't going well and eventually my mother had to meet with the teachers to discuss how to improve my marks. She remembers being in the teachers' lounge to discuss this difficult issue when someone jokingly suggested they pull out the Napoleon brandy. My mother and the teachers ultimately decided that I should drop French and use the time to concentrate on my other subjects. My French teacher was upset at this since he really liked me and believed I could excel in that language given time and help. However, my mother decided it was too much. Because I was now allowed to concentrate on my other subjects, I was able to improve my marks to a 60% average by Grade 12 and then finish Grade 13 with a 70% average.

I didn't make many friends in high school, although people accepted me and were generally nice. I just found it difficult to fit in, especially when Steve transferred to another school and I didn't have anyone to "break the ice" for me. But I did make another very good friend, Pierre, with whom I shared several common interests.

In my final year of high school, I joined the Outdoor Education Club and learned how to whitewater kayak. Since I was quite shy, the club helped bring me out of my shell. To this day, I wonder why I didn't join the club earlier even though I had been encouraged to do so. It wasn't until I became friends with Pierre, who was a member of the club, that I finally joined. Pierre and I have become great friends and we have had many memorable adventures together. He is a godparent to one of my children,

In 11th grade, my mother bought me a computer and I joined the school's computer club. That was the starting point of an important aspect of my life. Using a computer for my studies immediately improved my grammar. It helped me relate the words I typed to the words I read in books. It was also easier to make revisions in papers I wrote for school, which I did a lot. I had previously used a typewriter, a slow and frustrating process. Computers would later become the focus of my university education and career.

This stage of my life also marked the first time I earned an income. In 10th grade, I started a job delivering newspapers in my neighborhood. From Monday to Saturday, I had to get up at 5 a.m. to deliver the papers and followed that (except on Saturday) by going to school. This was an introduction to hard work and developing responsibility, and the income gave me some independence and flexibility.

As I think about the next chapter of my life, the following comes to mind: *What started out well didn't end well . . . but it wasn't the end of the world.*

In September of 1986, I entered Trent University in Peterborough, Ontario. I had applied to three universities and was accepted to each, but I chose Trent mainly because it was a small school and offered more opportunities for social interaction. I decided on a dual major in computer studies and history. The skills in communication I learned as a sailing instructor earlier that summer were extremely helpful the first few weeks at Trent. I became quite popular. In fact, on my birthday, I was surprised to walk out of my bedroom into a hallway full of streamers and balloons.

Nevertheless, my social life at school was challenging. The pubs were dark and very noisy, so it was always difficult to communicate. I was unable to lipread, which forced me to take paper and pen with me so I could communicate in writing if necessary. I didn't use that system too often with other men since "cheers" was usually all we needed to say. Women, however, seemed to find it very useful and I had several good conversations that way.

> Social life at school was challenging. The pubs were dark and noisy. It was difficult to communicate, so I would take paper and pen with me.

I made the Trent rowing team, but I must admit that rowing is very hard for a person who is deaf since it involves impeccable balance and timing. I wasn't able to hear it when the coxswain called out the order to speed up the stroke, so I constantly had to watch what my teammate in front of me was doing and react quickly to keep time. I really enjoyed the sport, and it was also through rowing that I met my first real girlfriend since childhood.

My first year at Trent was great. It was an entirely new experience, with new freedoms and the joy of meeting new people and trying different things. I played squash every week and even tried out for the ski team (which I failed to make). Unfortunately, all of these new experiences came at a cost since I neglected my studies. I completed only three subjects my first year and was put on probation for my second. It was strange going from a protected and limited environment at home to a university environment where you were responsible for yourself. I had to deal with increased awareness of my world and the responsibility that comes with it. I had to learn what it takes to meet and make friends. I had to deal with issues that I didn't need to worry about earlier in my life. It was an awakening. What had started at such a high level at the beginning of the school year had ended at such a low point the following spring. To make matters worse, my girlfriend broke up with me.

In the spring of 1987, I decided to go tree planting in northern Ontario. It was my first taste of hard work and was combined with a new experience in camping. I worked for two months in the early spring and then went to British

Columbia at the end of the summer to plant trees for a month. The work in British Columbia was really hard, but it was well worth it. I learned something that turned around my attitude about people. All year, I had endured periods when I felt lonesome, insecure, and even shy. Planting trees was difficult, and I would be so tired that I didn't even want to try to associate with my fellow planters. As a result, I blamed it on the others, believing that they didn't want to get to know me. I eventually learned that they really did want to get to know me. They just didn't know how to communicate with me and, therefore, left it up to me to bridge the gap. I realized then that if I were to have friends with normal hearing, I would have to take the first step.

The summer of 1987 was a difficult one for me because my parents decided to separate. In the fall, I went back to Trent University intending to socialize less and focus more on my studies. Almost immediately upon arriving, however, I fell in love with another girl. We didn't start dating until Christmas, but she broke up with me soon afterward, leaving me with a broken heart for about six months. I failed to make the rowing team that year, but

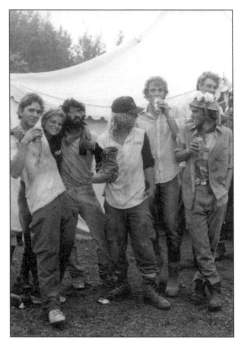

Here I am (far left) with friends I made while tree planting. The experience taught me that if I were to make friends with those with normal hearing, I would have to take the first step.

I did make the ski team, thanks to a new pair of skis. All in all, my second year turned out much better than my first, and I managed to complete five subjects.

I had notetakers for my classes at Trent. At first, I gave them carbon paper to work with, but because it proved such a hassle, I simply started photocopying their notes. I never had a problem finding notetakers since everyone was always so helpful. The seminars were another story, however. I never enjoyed them because I found it hard to keep track of who was speaking and what was being said. Consequently, I tried to avoid seminars whenever possible. The teachers were very understanding and would usually not mark against me for that.

In my third year at Trent, I met another wonderful woman. The problem was she already had a boyfriend, but I thought I would give it a try anyway. It didn't turn out the way I had hoped, but to this day we still keep in touch. Fortunately, I met another woman later in the school year and ended up dating her for nearly four years.

Finding a Career

When I finished at Trent in 1992, I started looking for my first full-time job. After searching for six months, I started working as a junior technical analyst at the Canadian Imperial Bank of Commerce (CIBC) in Toronto. I worked there for four years, advancing eventually to the position of senior technical analyst. It was a very good job and gave me exposure to the working world. Plus, the people with whom I worked were great. In 1996, however, I left CIBC to pursue another dream of mine: to ride a bicycle around New Zealand.

Steve and I cycled more than 3,000 kilometers in two months and had a great time. I then returned to Canada and spent the rest of the summer painting at my parents' cottage. In October, I began to search for a new career, and in January, I accepted a position at the accounting firm of Ernst & Young in Toronto. I have been there since. In fact, after only six months at Ernst & Young, I had moved up into Technical Services, the design and engineering department for information technology.

People often ask if my deafness has been a barrier to progress. My answer is both yes and no. My deafness narrows the number of opportunities I can get. For example, I can't work in call center services because it involves using the phone. To hire me, an employer will have to determine, "Where can Richard work so his deafness will not be a factor?" That is usually in areas where typical interaction with users is not required, areas usually found at the higher levels of information technology. Thus, even though I can't do certain things, it ironically forces me into areas that are more challenging, very interesting, and highly enjoyable. I have a very good work ethic. Given an opportunity, I do my best to prove myself.

The Pros and Cons of Being Deaf

I wear hearing aids, which helps, but it doesn't substitute for normal hearing. Being deaf, however, does have its rewards. Not being able to hear a baby crying at night and always getting a good night's sleep can be an advantage. On the other hand, it can be a shock to feel your wife poking you and telling you to get up to check the baby.

Another prime example is what happened to me when I was cycling around New Zealand with Steve. After a long, tiring day, we camped beside a beautiful river not far from a railroad bridge. It was quiet and peaceful. We had dinner, pitched the tent, and climbed into our sleeping bags for a good night's rest. At 4 in the morning, Steve forcibly woke me up and I, thinking something was seriously wrong, exclaimed, "What's going on?" He had a jealous look on his face and asked if I knew what was happening. "No," I replied. "Go back to sleep." He kicked me again and told me that trains had been going by every 20 minutes with their horns blowing; plus, a bird had been relentlessly attacking the outside of the tent. Needless to say, poor Steve didn't get much sleep that night.

Being deaf can be good in some ways, but dangerous in others, especially when warnings cannot be heard. When I was 4 years old, I had an accident that could have permanently scarred me. I was at my aunt's house playing near her swimming pool when I saw behind a glass door two lovely Afghan hounds that I wanted to pet. What I didn't know was that they were barking. I couldn't hear them. When I opened the door, they jumped on me and tore my face to shreds. I was rushed to the hospital and received 45 stitches.

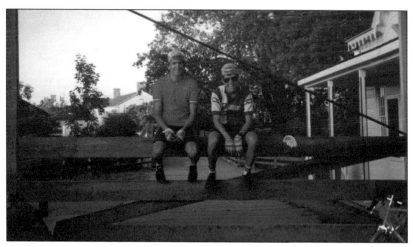

Steve (right) and I take a break en route to Quebec City from Toronto in 1984, one of our many cycling trips.

Fortunately, I was very young and healed with no scars. Despite the accident with the dogs, I never lost my love of animals, and at one point even considered making a career of veterinary medicine. Today, I own a lovely yellow Labrador.

When I was growing up, language and vocabulary had to be taught directly to most children who were deaf. Those were different times, and it was very difficult — in fact, almost impossible — for a young child with hearing loss to learn language spontaneously outside therapy. In second grade, I came home from school once and proudly blurted an expletive to my mother. She was so pleased, she hugged and congratulated me. To which my brother complained, "Well, when I swear, I get my mouth washed out with soap." The reason my mother was so happy was because these were the first words I had learned off the street — outside my daily therapy program. My parents remember saying words such as "ball" to me about ten thousand times before I finally said something similar. With my daughter Scarlett, I only need to say a word two or three times before she can repeat it, which amazes me.

Steve believes that because I usually can't overhear what people say, I'm a perfect example of the "water off a duck's back" analogy, meaning words don't affect me as they should and I have an easier time letting go of comments others may make. Since I cannot hear well, my friends believe that I have too much faith in people — that I am not as judgmental because I can't overhear what some people say about others. People are also able to talk about me right in front of me. I remember an old girlfriend organizing a surprise birthday party for me on the phone when I was right in the room.

My upbringing had a great impact on my family. My father and brother didn't get as much attention from my mother so they would devise ways to grab some. My brother, for instance, needed to wear foot braces as a child when he was sleeping. When we had company in the house, he would wait in his bedroom until the braces were on and then hobble downstairs in front of everybody. Jamey told me recently that he suffered a condition as a child that no one at the time knew about: delayed metalinguistic development, which is the inability to learn the sounds of the alphabet. He didn't realize this issue until his wife, a speech pathologist, noticed it in one of their children. Perhaps my parents didn't pick up on it because they were so busy with me or, compared to my situation, they didn't realize its significance. My brother feels that he became a stronger and more independent person because of all this.

My father also had a proactive role in ensuring that I would be in the same sports programs as Jamey, and the only way to do that was to run many of the programs himself. Some of the other coaches, it seems, didn't want me on their teams. Therefore, he coached my hockey team, my football team, and even managed the Nancy Green ski team despite not knowing how to ski.

The most important influence in my life, however, was my mother. There is no way I would be where I am today if she hadn't made exceptional efforts on my behalf. She was always there for me, diligently working with me day after day to ensure that I progressed at an appropriate level. She always provided support and encouragement. She always made the effort to teach people how to interact with me.

> My father had a proactive role in ensuring I'd be in the same sports programs as my brother Jamey: He ran many of the programs himself.

An example of her determination in ensuring that I would be integrated into the hearing community was when I entered first grade. Administrators at the school wanted the school psychologist to test me; however, the last thing my mother wanted was for them to find out the degree of my hearing loss since she had heard from a friend that the psychologist had suggested that "all deaf children should be sent to a special school." My mother told the school that I had a little bit of a hearing problem, but because I had been through so many tests already, it wasn't necessary to test me again. Unbelievably, the school officials agreed with her and allowed me in. In sixth grade, I was accidentally tested and they were horrified to learn how severe my hearing loss was. By then, however, it wasn't an issue.

My mother met the teachers before the start of each semester and told them, "It's not your fault if it doesn't work out; just do your best." She kept a notepad for daily correspondence with the teachers. The notebook would contain information such as what we were going to do in class the next day and questions such as "How did I do in school that day?" and "What areas do I need to work on?" Every morning, before she went to work, my mother spent an hour with me on my speech and school lessons. She continued to do this until 10th grade when she could no longer understand the math. We continued to do speech work two or three times a week until I entered Trent University. I also went for weekly speech therapy until my third year at Trent.

A Family of My Own

It was at my father's wedding reception in April of 1993 that I met Sarah, who would become my wife. She was working behind the bar and I knew as soon as I saw her that I would marry her one day. Surprisingly, I knew instantly that she wasn't from Canada since her lip movements were different and often very challenging. It turned out she was British. I called her up the next day using the Bell Canada Relay service and we talked for an hour. What struck me was that she wasn't *embarrassed* communicating with me through a third party on the phone, which some people find uncomfortable. We went on our first date several days later and she moved in with me about 3 months later. Later that year, she returned to England to begin her university program in marketing. We maintained a long-distance relationship for 5 years before marrying in June of 1998. I think in some ways that my perseverance helped to keep our relationship together. Meeting all her family and friends with all their regional British accents certainly put my lipreading skills to the test.

The first addition to the family was a wonderful yellow Labrador in the summer of 2000. Our first child, Scarlett, was born in August 2001, and our second child, Ruby, was born in October 2003.

I never fully realized the difficulty my parents must have gone through when I was a child until Scarlett and Ruby were born. I was extra conscious of the fact that my children might have a hearing loss even though there was no biological or genetic reason to suspect they would. My children's hearing was tested when each was a few months old, with positive results. It amazes me that Scarlett and Ruby will wake up when they hear me walking up the stairs, or stop crying when I call their names. I can't imagine how my parents coped with my situation.

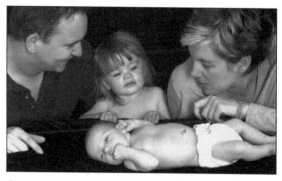

It amazes me that our daughters Scarlett and Ruby will wake up when they hear me walking up the stairs. I can't imagine how my parents coped with my hearing loss.

Adapting Just Fine

I'm often asked if I know what caused my deafness. All I can I say is that I don't know — no one really knows. When my mom was ill early in her pregnancy, she was given an antibiotic that has been known in some cases to cause deafness. As you recall, I was born premature. I experienced apnea spells while in intensive care as a newborn, and my heart stopped that time in the nursery. I don't think any of these events alone caused my deafness because hearing is supposed to be fully developed by the third trimester, which is about 28 weeks. I was 28 weeks old when I was born, so in theory my hearing should have been fully developed.

I have adapted to my hearing loss extremely well, but I will deal with it for the rest of my life. I am a functioning member of society, thanks to a combination of Auditory-Verbal therapy and the support of my wonderful family and many dear friends. I don't regret not being able to hear normally. I don't even see it as a disability. Understandably, it was an issue during my teenage and university years when I faced an unknown future. But now, in my mid-30s, it isn't an issue. My wife finds it frustrating that she can't just talk to me when she is in the middle of something. She has to stop what she's doing, or she has to find me if I'm in another room, so I can read her lips. However, we deal with it.

I am interested in having cochlear implant surgery, but at the moment it is not as important since my hearing has been stable for several years. Maybe if it gets worse, I will consider having the surgery. For the moment, I remain content with my hearing aids. Of course, if one of my children were deaf, I would seriously consider having her fitted for an implant and would begin Auditory-Verbal therapy as soon as possible.

Thoughts on Growing Up Deaf

Because of my experiences, I've adopted the following list of advice:

- Don't worry too much about issues you can't control. For example, don't feel bad if you don't hear someone say "Hello" and when you don't respond that person thinks you're rude. He or she will get to know you eventually, find out what an amazing person you are, and understand then why you didn't respond that first time.

- Don't be afraid to ask people to repeat themselves, and don't feel bad if they ask you to repeat yourself. It's a two-way street. We all want to communicate.

- Life is about how you feel. If you constantly worry how other people perceive you because of your deafness, you won't be happy. It is extremely important that you focus on what makes you happy. If something doesn't make you happy, then change it or don't do it. You may not be as popular as you would like, but you will feel happier, satisfied, and more content with yourself.

- Don't hold yourself back. Always try something at least more than once, and if you still don't like it, well, at least you tried. You will be surprised at how much you can do.

- Family support is extremely important, and there must be a dedicated adult who is committed to working with you.

- Immersion in hearing activities is extremely important in developing friends and being confident you can cope in the hearing world.

- Talk about your needs with stakeholders, such as peers and teachers.

- Take the "e" out of emotion when there is a problem. Do something about it.

- Give at least 20 minutes a day to your immediate family members.

- Goals are very important to help keep your focus.

- Find or create a parental support group.

- Research the latest therapy techniques in Auditory-Verbal therapy and technology.

- Never be afraid to ask for help.

- Read everything you can.

Conclusion

In 2003, I achieved one of my long-term goals when I completed my master's degree in information technology. I achieved my degree on the Internet, and it offered a powerful insight on how well deaf people can do if they are provided the appropriate learning medium. Before this experience, education for me was mostly sitting in a hearing classroom and lipreading what the teachers said as much as possible. I had to rely on notetakers, but I feel I ultimately educated myself. The onus was on me to teach myself and learn since no one was going to do it for me. If I wanted to survive, I had to find a way to cope in the hearing world. True, my family, friends, and many teachers did their best to help me, but I mostly had to learn how to teach myself. As a result, I have an enormous ability for self-learning and comprehension of information. So, when online courses became a reality, I no longer had to rely on my lipreading skills since all of the material was text-based. I was surprised at how well I did in my master's program. In fact, I received better marks than in any course I had taken in the classroom.

Individuals who are deaf can do very well in the hearing world if they are offered the appropriate communication tools. Technology such as e-mail and the interactive pager has helped bridge the gap between those who can hear and those who don't. Being deaf means having to become independent and working harder to earn the respect of colleagues, especially those with normal hearing. We have to go the extra mile and demonstrate integrity in what we do. We must achieve a high level of education. We offer skills to those in the working world such as patience and the ability to focus — skills that many with normal hearing do not perform as well as we do.

Being deaf in a hearing world can be a great asset. After all, we aren't interrupted as often as hearing people.

I never tried to hold back when opportunities appeared. If I had a chance to learn a new skill or sport, then I would try to figure out how I could do it. It was very important to have goals since they gave me a sense of direction and purpose.

I am proud of myself and am proud to be deaf. I welcome the challenges it offers. I never look at the negative aspects of my hearing loss, only the positive and how I can use them to my advantage.

I started this story with a quote from 1973 that I found while looking over my mother's records. I knew the quote was important to her because she had underlined it, and it obviously set the stage for her mission in raising me. Thirty-one years later, I'm happy to prove how significant her influence on me was.

CHAPTER 6

Vanessa

Vanessa Vaughan

I was born in November 1969, the year Neil Armstrong and Buzz Aldrin walked on the moon. As a child, I persistently asked if I could fly to the moon myself one day, to which my mother would reply with a simple, "Possibly." Thankfully, my parents always helped me feel I could do anything, a sentiment I now share with my own child.

My daughter Stella had her hearing tested on the third day of her life. I realize how fortunate we are today that so much progress has been made in technology and the sharing of information. Parents can now find out very early whether their child has a health risk that might need immediate attention. When Stella was born, I walked away from the hospital with pamphlets filled with hearing-related information, aware that hearing loss today can be detected at birth. It saves so much time in this world of uncertainty. After all, the baby is unable tell you. You cannot see deafness.

My mother was present for Stella's hearing test. It was a gift having her there. More than 30 years ago, she was one of the pioneering activists of VOICE for Hearing Impaired Children (VOICE), an organization whose mandate was to lobby for early hearing screening for newborns and infants. Stella's test was completed in almost no time, before we left the hospital. It was a moment for which my mother had been waiting a long time.

Early Signs of Trouble

There is no known history of deafness in my family. I appeared normal in every way, but it didn't take long for my parents to begin wondering whether I had a problem since I wasn't as responsive as other babies. My mother had had a very healthy pregnancy with me. I weighed 6½ pounds and arrived full term. Since everything seemed normal, it never occurred to my parents to get my hearing checked early.

I have no memory of sound, but I do remember being enveloped in warmth and stillness and seeing many vibrant things. I also recall the enjoyable sensation of floating when I was being carried around.

I had a deep sense of safety. I recall being held in my father's arms, looking up into his eyes. Perhaps because I didn't hear, I was more sensitive to energy and a kind of astral projection, to connect with others and make sense of many situations.

Our house was rich in color and texture, and I recall being mesmerized by many patterns, in particular light patterns radiating from the colorful stained-glass windows in the living room where I often played. I was captivated, and sitting there felt timeless. I became very aware of light and was intrigued by how the colors changed as the sun passed by the window. I spent hours staring at the window as the vivid light flickered through the leaves blowing in the wind. It was music for the eyes.

I'm told I was a normal, jovial baby — alert and absorbed in play. I recall seeing a man walk through the doorway of our home day after day, pass the living room where I was, wave his hand, and then disappear. This man with smiling eyes, with the same wave even to this day, turned out to be my father. Some days I happened to see him, but on others I didn't look up to the sound of his voice. I appeared disinterested. Seeing him regularly became a rhythm of comfort. He came home at the end of the day to say, "Hello, Vanessa. How are you?" But I wouldn't respond. I just kept doing what I was doing.

After a while, my mother began to think it was strange I wasn't more responsive to my father's routine. She speculated that I was exhibiting behaviors similar to children with autism.

My mother watched as other infants my age babbled and played with their voices far more than I did. For example, I wouldn't follow directions, and I wouldn't respond. Unlike Lisa and Kelly, the neighborhood children who were born within a month of me, I wasn't babbling. I loved to play with Lisa and Kelly, but I was noticeably quiet. We developed a telepathic type of play language, and through the years we understood what we were thinking without saying a word.

It seemed I was inside my own little bubble of warmth and security — a world of stillness where I was comfortable being alone, swaddled in a blanket of silence. This positive sense of solitude is how I came to know life.

As my mother would say later:

> *"I know in the beginning Vanessa made many sounds. There was cooing and baby sounds that indicated to me that she was fine. It never even occurred to me that there was anything amiss. Then the noises stopped. Around the same time, she began to scream so loudly . . . in a very high-pitched voice. I realize now that she couldn't even hear the tone or the level of her voice."*

My mother was a sensitive and intuitive person. She knew something wasn't quite right with her first-born child, but she wasn't really sure what to do.

Diagnosis and Disbelief

I owe the discovery of my hearing loss to my great aunt Dianne, who often babysat me. She noticed one day that I didn't even flinch to the loud ringing of our kitchen phone when I was right beside it. It dawned on her that I might be deaf. She brought out all types of kitchen gadgets and banged away at them as I sat there, but I didn't respond. At that moment, she said, a lump went from her throat right through her soul and worked its way into my parents' hearts. When she told my parents what had happened, they were spurred to take me to an ENT specialist at the Hospital for Sick Children in Toronto.

At the hospital, I was put in a dimly lit, beige clinical booth and placed before a board with a number of colored pegs. I remember a blonde lady working with me. When she put a yellow peg into one of the holes on the board, I did the same, and then copied her again when she placed a red peg in another hole. Either I was obsessed with copying or had intuitive psychic abilities about what was expected of me.

The ENT specialist told my mother that I could hear just fine, but it turned out that I was just a highly observant child. My mother remained convinced that something wasn't right, however, and finally decided to take me to see some psychology students at the Ontario Institute for Studies in Education, the Toronto educational facility where she worked. They spent the whole afternoon playing with me and solved the mystery. Just as my great aunt had suspected, they confirmed that everything was all right except I couldn't hear anything.

When they heard the news, my parents had no clue what steps to take first. My father was determined to find out everything he could, but my mother was simply confused. She blamed herself, but wasn't sure exactly why. She had yet to meet anyone with a hearing loss.

Without delay, my parents underwent genetic testing and counseling. The test results, however, indicated that my deafness wasn't hereditary. Hearing aids were prescribed, but my mother thought all she had to do was put them on me and I would hear. She wasn't prepared for the resulting shock and despair when that didn't happen.

My mother's feeling of helplessness continued, but then Louise Crawford from the Hospital for Sick Children called and offered to train me auditorially. We met within a week of her call, beginning a relationship of weekly sessions that would last nearly 10 years. We still keep in touch today.

My mother, who had a background in education, began visiting schools for the deaf in the Toronto area. She was dismayed by the lack of communication in the classrooms between children and their teachers. She also noticed that the sign language used in the early 1970s by the teachers and students was inconsistent, meaning communication was confusing and a continuous problem.

The language barrier in the schools for the deaf was one of the main reasons my mother decided to enroll me in the neighborhood school, which conveniently faced the backyard of our home and had a playground I could see through our garden fence. She wanted me to be part of the local community and thought it would be easier for me to be part of an English-speaking world than one in which everyone used sign language.

> My mother thought it would be easier for me to be part of an English-speaking world than one in which everyone used sign language.

Striving for Normalcy

I have two younger brothers. Ben was born a year-and-a-half after me, and Zach came six-and-a-half years after Ben. It never really occurred to them that I was different. They figured deafness was just a part of life.

At first, I neither understood the concept that Ben was my brother nor why he was even there with us. I was only beginning to understand abstract ideas. The first time my mother was away from home was when she went to the hospital to deliver Ben. I knew that something big was in the air. I knew he was someone special since I felt so much joy every time I was taken to his crib to have a peek.

One day, as a young child, Ben joined my mother at a VOICE meeting (without me so he could have a chance to feel important and special). Ben had told my itinerant teacher that he thought his sister was lucky to be deaf because she was able to go to all the fun places, such as conferences, panel meetings, parent groups for children with hearing loss, and therapy.

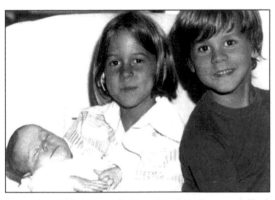

It never really occurred to my brothers Ben and Zach (in my arms) that I was different. They figured deafness was just a part of life.

Ben would never admit it, but I know he felt left out. He spent hours sitting under the table playing with his toys, yelling out the right answers as my mother and I did speech drills and listening exercises. She often ignored him unintentionally while focusing on the auditory lessons, but I never heard him shout out the answers. Now I understand why he is so smart. I also know why he grew up more independent than most children and was so ahead of his classmates. He was constantly immersed in language and exposed to many experiences, including the gallery of language pictures that were found in every corner of our house.

Ben often did presentations at school about sound and hearing aids. One of his roommates at university wrote her thesis on deaf and hard of hearing issues and came to interview me, an indication that Ben shared a lot outside the home about his experiences with a sister who is deaf.

My brother Zach and I are very close. He arrived after the rigorous auditory training years, so we had time for a more typical sibling relationship. I was also old enough to babysit him as we grew up. Both Ben and Zach turned out to be sensitive men, always making sure I didn't feel left out of conversations during family functions.

My grandfather's response to my deafness was to assist the family any way possible. He offered to help my parents send me away to a boarding school for the deaf. My mother, however, didn't want to send me away, thinking it was best for me to be close to home. I was to have as normal a childhood as possible. She was determined to help me overcome the obstacles of being deaf in a hearing world.

I have an uncle with special needs, the youngest of seven children. He lived in a home for the mentally challenged and was never around for family functions. For many years, I wondered if this was one of the reasons the relationship between my mother and her parents-in-law was strained. Perhaps my mother felt I was being rejected as an imperfect child, too. However, that was the mindset of my grandparents' generation. Parents were simply told by "experts" what to do for their child with special needs and that's what they did — just as my grandparents did with my uncle.

From a very young age, I had a strong connection with my grandmothers. They lived in the same neighborhood; therefore, I had the luxury of seeing them regularly. They always helped me feel special since I was their brown-eyed princess.

One of my grandmothers, Gammy, spent a lot of time reading, playing the piano, and watching me paint and draw. She worked at the complaints department of a large department store and would bring home all types of returned clothing. Using her sewing wizardry, Gammy and my mother would add pockets to everything for my big, metal hearing aids. Gammy and I would also watch "Tiny Talent Time" on television, enjoying the performances of the children. It was one of the only TV shows I could understand fully before closed captioning arrived. Therefore, I loved to dress up and dance and pretend I was on television, too.

My other grandmother, Dodee, was one of Canada's first female pilots and constantly told me to follow my dreams. She stressed that if I set my mind to it I would be able to accomplish what my heart desired. She abandoned her interest in aviation to start a family and ended up raising seven children.

Many years later, I went on to write, produce, and direct an internationally broadcast short film dedicated to my grandmothers. *Edda's Song* was about two women from different generations who met in a park and realized it is never too late to follow your dreams.

Despite my deafness, I related to both my grandmothers very well. They treated me as they treated everyone else, instilling in me the confidence to pursue dreams and celebrate uniqueness.

I asked my mother if she remembered how other people reacted to my hearing loss and she said, "I was way too busy to even think about what other people thought, and could not have cared less!" She pointed out that she was also running a rooming house and was pregnant with my brother at the time.

'The Olfactory Period'

Like Picasso, who went through different stages of painting (such as his famous Blue Period), I refer to my childhood years as the "Olfactory Period," since my sense of smell was so strong.

Assorted aromas hovered around my childhood adventures: the warm smell of flour, bread, and date cookies . . . the potent scents of the lilac trees,

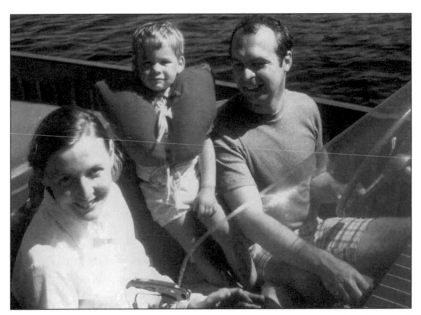

As a child I played in water a lot. I would swim underwater and blow bubbles. I would exclaim, "I can hear! I can hear!" Years later, I created a painting titled "I Heard the Bubbles Singing," which now hangs in a collector's home.

lily of the valley, and peonies in our magical garden . . . the stench of wet sand at the cottage . . . the stale odor of museums . . . the smokiness emanating from the walls in my grandparents' home.

Back then, I was lucky to have my mother by my side most of the time. After she worked to put my father through school, my parents decided she would leave the work force and stay home with the kids, which she did until Zach was old enough to attend school all day. She offered us a wealth of creative play, aided by her careers as an English and drama teacher and a newspaper reporter. I spent hours with my mother being bathed in language. I find I am doing the same with Stella even though she isn't deaf.

My mother and I did a lot of cooking and baking together and I was immersed in language. It was a great way to learn numbers, measurements, ingredients, and temperatures. I continue to love food experimentation and culinary delights.

Despite the silence, my childhood was a feast of sight, color, and taste, which led to my appreciation of art, nature, and food. Scents rather than sounds still trigger bountiful memories and a multitude of emotions.

The best way to describe what I was sensing was that I was very aware of energy, body language, and facial expressions. That is why I believe Lisa and I communicated telepathically. We had invented our own little language.

I remember playing in water a lot. I loved splashing around and loved the soothing silky sensation of swimming. Every year at the summer cottage, I would jump into the lake, swim underwater, and blow bubbles. The vibration of blowing bubbles underwater made a sound in my ears and I would exclaim, "I can hear! I can hear!" Years later, I created a painting titled "I Heard the Bubbles Singing," which now hangs in a collector's home.

Sharing a Love of Music

My mother has a degree in music and is an accomplished pianist. She also taught steel pan drumming and once was invited to perform in Toronto's Caribana Parade. Since both my parents were musical, they were sad they were unable to share their love of music with me.

Still, they tried. One of my favorite memories is of my mother strumming the guitar, wearing her bell-bottom jeans, singing songs to Ben and me as we lounged on the floor.

She encouraged Ben and me to learn to play the piano, so we took lessons for years. She believed that playing an instrument would help me develop intonation and pitch, and improve the quality of my voice. I loved playing the piano, though I did grumble about practicing.

Now that I have a cochlear implant, my husband Jonathan enjoys sharing his love for the Grateful Dead. He took me to my first concert, in fact, to hear the soothing acoustics of Jerry Garcia.

The Benefits of Auditory Training

As I mentioned above, my parents were referred to Louise Crawford when I was about 15 months old. Miss Crawford wanted to begin therapy immediately, just as the summer was beginning, but I didn't have my first auditory training session until the fall when I was 18 months old. Little did my parents know that in those three months between diagnosis and initiation of therapy a critical window for language acquisition had passed. Valuable time had been lost.

We would see Miss Crawford once a week, but she also would provide therapy ideas for my mother to work on daily at home. Our therapy sessions took place right after her lunch hour and I remember seeing her from the waiting room, without fail, carrying her toothbrush down the hall. This was a signal that I was to go in shortly.

Miss Crawford had many stuffed animals and toys in her office, which we played with to learn vowel sounds. I still have some of those toys tucked away in a metal travel box. It has become a treasure chest of memories for me.

To develop listening skills with my minimal residual hearing, Miss Crawford, in one exercise, would stand at the back of the room behind me and ask questions. I was unable to see her and it was extremely difficult to understand a word this way. I would strain very hard to heighten my psychic abilities to see whether I could catch a word correctly, without lipreading. As I got older, I discovered a trick. My metal hearing aid acted like a mirror. I would hold it in such a way that I could see the reflection of her face. I wonder if she ever knew what I was doing. At the time, I was proud of myself for discovering this communication technique. Not only could I lipread backward but also far away at the same time.

Miss Crawford was very proper. In her formal, highly structured lessons, I learned etiquette such as being polite and not interrupting while others were talking. I learned to sit still, to focus and be disciplined.

As a 5-year-old, I was a subject in the Canadian Broadcasting Corporation documentary *The Children Who Learned to Listen,* hosted by David Suzuki. In the documentary, which showed what children in Auditory-Verbal therapy could achieve, I was filmed responding to questions asked by Miss Crawford. Looking back, I am amazed by the words I knew at the age of 5, such as *daily* and *creature,* and by the kind of questions I could answer, such as "What do you do daily?"

I remember staring at the camera lens, intrigued by the moving iris. I knew one day I would be back in front of the camera. It was then I realized that I must be doing something important to have visitors take such an interest in me with a fancy apparatus. It was an ego boost!

The CBC experience also planted the acting seed for me during my youth. When I was 10, I auditioned for a movie called *Clown White.* The casting director called Miss Crawford for a referral, that turned out to be me. The director said he liked being able to talk to me since he didn't know sign language. I got the part, along with another student, because I could speak and listen and understand the spoken directions from the filmmakers (unlike some of the other kids who auditioned who primarily used sign language). The cast included a mix of children who were both aural deaf and hard of hearing. On the set, I learned the sign language alphabet for the first time and became intrigued with it. But I also experienced feelings of inadequacy because the kids who were signing couldn't understand me.

A scene I had in another movie, *Crazy Moon* (starring Kiefer Sutherland), reminded me of my own experiences growing up. After months and months of silence, my first word was "aaaahhhh" (for airplane). I was sitting in the back seat of my parents' car, looking out the window, when I saw an airplane and said it. My parents were literally so excited that they slammed on their brakes in the middle of the highway. That's kind of what happened in *Crazy Moon,* when a family gets very excited about my character (Anne) being able to say "carrrr-buuuuraaator" (for carburetor). Doing that scene was very emotional for me. Watching the actors who were playing my parents, I could empathize with how my mother and father must have felt when I finally showed them I was ready to learn to talk.

An Extra Year of Preschool

I attended a nursery school where there was a lot of music and painting, and I went there for an extra year instead of going directly to kindergarten. My mother thought it was better if I continued in a familiar environment, and she even joined me at the school for the first few months to help the teacher work one-on-one with the students. She then volunteered from time to time to keep tabs on me. I remember her watching me in music class as we danced around the room moving like horses, elephants, and giraffes.

I didn't really begin to talk for a long time, and my speech was unintelligible to anyone outside my immediate family. I only started to say a few words during my second year of nursery school. I loved dancing during music classes but didn't interact verbally with other kids. It was only through physical play that I was able to fit in. I was a good runner and great at playing tag. I could see everything that was going on. I didn't feel any different from the other children.

I went with the flow and spent time observing others in the school yard, unable to hear the sounds that typically accompanied children at play. I learned games simply by copying others and filling in gaps through observation. I didn't always understand what was happening or completely comprehend the reality of my situation. I thought the feelings I experienced were normal and that everyone was in the same boat. The other children were interacting a lot more than I realized.

At my nursery school, there was a guardian angel always on watch by the name of Ms. Taylor, a tall and vibrant woman with very black and expressive, twinkling eyes. Without fail, she said good morning to me every single day even though I didn't respond until my second year there. The first time I said good morning back to her, she immediately called my mother to let her know. It turned out to be big news.

What I remember most about nursery school was doing art. I loved the painting easels, colorful jars, and big brushes. I loved immersing my fingers in the paint and moving them as though part of a dance onto the paper. Painting gave me confidence. It was the one thing I did that I could fully claim as my own.

At home, I spent hours sitting on my mother's lap as she drew all kinds of pictures in an attempt to explain abstract concepts. *Daddy is going to the office* consisted of a picture of a stick figure walking to a car, driving the car, walking to a building, and, lastly, sitting behind a desk. We had pictures all over the house, and sometimes it took forever to go upstairs or downstairs as we paused on each step to discuss the pictures.

The Jump to Kindergarten

Because I was just starting to open up, my mother thought the extra year in nursery school would be beneficial. My friend Lisa had moved on to the "big school" and kindergarten, but we waited.

French Immersion classes were being introduced and becoming popular about the time I started kindergarten. However, it was hard enough for me to learn spoken English, so I didn't go into French Immersion like Lisa and my brother, along with a couple of other playmates from my neighborhood. That was about the time it started to sink in that there was something different or special about me.

My kindergarten teacher's class was a mecca for play. There was an indoor sandbox and baby chickens in a large aluminum cage. I got my finger trapped in the hatching cage once and hurt it badly. I cried a lot and only later discovered that I had not heard my teacher give explicit instructions about how to handle the cage. The other kids appeared to have told me I was wrong, and I felt as though I had done something bad . . . more clues that I was different.

I loved being in motion. I remember running out toward the swings as soon as the recess door opened. I don't remember interacting with a lot of kids, but

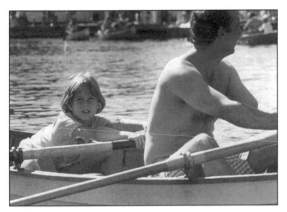

When I was a child, I loved being in motion. About the time this photo was taken, I began to receive itinerant hearing support services and used an FM system for the first time.

my verbal skills came alive as I started to talk to the teacher without knowing what other kids were saying or whether someone else was speaking. I spent time observing people and wondering about their lives, families, and homes. I imagined stories about everyone and everything around me.

Finding My Way in Elementary School

My elementary school was located just around the corner on the same block, so I could walk to it every day. Still, it seemed like a huge schlep. I now wonder if the world for children who are deaf is even smaller than for "hearing" children of the same age when it comes to their physical relationship to life.

My first-grade teacher, Mr. Smyke, was a towering man of great stature who introduced the class to the reading series *Mr. Mugs*, about a beloved sheepdog. I could follow along pretty well since I had learned how to read early and was initially ahead of the class in this area. To help me keep up, my mother would come to the classroom to assist the teacher. I discovered the real reason she came much later.

It wasn't until first or second grade, when I was about 6, that my speech started to become more intelligible to those outside my family. I started to talk a lot more, and I interrupted in class because I wasn't hearing other students talking. Mr. Smyke taught me the importance of not interrupting and how to carefully take note of my surroundings.

In second grade, I moved downstairs to Miss Millwood's class, where I also stayed for third grade. One day, she asked the class to come up with words that have "art" in them, such as *cart, mart*, and *smart*. Without knowing what it meant, I wrote in the word *fart*, having gone down the alphabet trying to create new words. When I finally figured out its meaning, I was embarrassed for days. Learning impolite words was very important because I didn't naturally pick them up by overhearing other children's chatter.

In fourth grade, I had to deliver a lot of oral presentations, which caused me a great deal of stress. One boy in the class constantly made fun of me, and whenever I got up for a presentation he would make faces and contort his lips. For many years after that, I felt self-conscious about my speech.

In fifth grade, I began to receive itinerant hearing support services, although I had been using an FM system for a couple of years. After my first meeting with my itinerant teacher, Joan, I asked, "Do I have to come again?" and "Does my mother know about this?" Little did I know she would be my itinerant teacher for many years. She taught me the importance of being on time and the art of beautiful penmanship.

I was always determined to sit in the back of the classroom. I was more comfortable there since it helped me feel in control of my environment — like a watchdog or a fighter pilot; a place where I could navigate all the action and be on top of things. This horrified my itinerant teacher, who immediately arranged to have me moved up to the front. I hated being there. Not hearing or seeing what was going on behind me made me very uncomfortable and uncertain.

The thinking at that time was that students who are deaf or hard of hearing should sit in the front in mainstreamed classrooms. There were several reasons for this. Before the advent of FM systems, the student needed to be as close as possible to the teacher in order to hear. Hearing aids were most effective when the speaker's voice was 6–8 inches from the microphone — a challenge in any classroom! With the pupil with hearing loss sitting "front and center," the teacher would be reminded of his or her presence and would, hopefully, remember to follow key teaching strategies: not moving around too much during the lesson; writing significant words or points on the blackboard (but not talking with his or her back to the class); speaking naturally but as clearly as possible; ensuring that the light fell on the teacher's face rather than coming from behind; and so forth.

Best of Friends

My friend Lisa played a major role throughout my life. She taught me to be street smart, encouraged me to develop uniqueness through my art, taught me about relationships, and generally shared what life was all about. She was the friend who held my social tapestry together.

Once, Lisa and I set up a flower shop on the front lawn. We cut all the beautiful tulips around us and put them on display on little tables. We were so proud of our entrepreneurial spirit, and only later did I realize that Lisa's mother had warned us from inside the house not to cut the flowers. I didn't hear her, but Lisa did. Her father returned from work raving mad. I didn't understand why he was so angry and couldn't read his furiously moving lips. By that time, I was aware of the limitations of my hearing, and learned that if I didn't pay attention I could get into plenty of trouble.

Lisa and I could see each other from our bedroom windows since our houses were side by side. Each night, we waved good night to each other, and would peer out the window the following morning to see if the other was up. We would press pictures we had drawn against the window panes and decide who had drawn the better picture of a tree or flower. We also chatted from our windows by lipreading and miming. Lisa, who has perfect hearing, learned to lipread by growing up with me.

When we were older, we traveled for a few months to Paris and shared a tiny apartment, perfect roommates the entire time. Lisa was a night owl to the extreme. All I had to do was take off my hearing aids when I went to sleep and she could play her music loudly and roam about painting well into the wee hours of the morning. We would spend hours together and not speak. We were comfortable in our shared silence, with Lisa relishing the freedom that gave her. Whenever we talked, however, the conversations always had profound significance.

As an artist, Lisa lived all over the world: Florence, Paris, Berlin. But even in times where the distance between us was great, we remained connected. I am sad to say that Lisa died recently of breast cancer. The world is less colorful in her absence.

High School: A Time to Bond

I faced additional challenges in high school when phone conversations became a big thing. In my house, we had two black dial phones side by side and my mother would interpret all the calls for me. This made my friends nervous and hesitant to call. According to my mother, my girlfriends wanted to talk for hours about nothing, which bored her to tears. They were also dying to talk about boys, yet they were afraid to do so with a parent screening the calls. Thank goodness for e-mail today. My 12-year-old goddaughter, who is deaf, walks around with a two-way e-mail pager.

High school was very cliquey, and I didn't belong to any particular group. I would weave in and out of groups as a free agent. I actually preferred it that way because it allowed me to have more quality one-on-one friendships. It also made me feel proud to celebrate individualism with those to whom I gravitated through common interests such as art and film. It was easier for me to communicate that way and to keep up with the gossip. Fast-paced conversations in large groups were both hard to follow and stressful.

I had some very special hearing "big sister" friends who were a little older than me. They were my role models and helped me keep up with what was cool. They babysat me and took me shopping or to the movies. One of these big sisters, Ruth, still supports me as I continue to explore motherhood.

My mother always arranged for me to get together with older girls who were deaf, and I grew to admire them. I loved getting together with Frances (whose story also is in this book) and Sarah Jane. I looked up to them as independent and strong girls who understood the trials and tribulations of being mainstreamed. When I did things with them, I could be myself and relax. I wasn't concerned about speaking clearly and, as a result, conversation flowed more easily. Time with them as a young girl and teenager was very special. It allowed me to see that everything was going to be all right when I grew up.

In ninth grade, I met a girl named Janet with whom I became very close. She and I would write long letters to each other every night and pop the letters into each other's locker. Each morning, I would arrive at school eager to read about the crush of the day and all of the previous day's gossip. Today, of course, kids have cell phones and two-way pagers to keep current.

Back then, an important activity for me was our time spent in the "Saturday Night Club." The club was started by local teenagers who were deaf or hard of hearing who decided, after a taxing week at a mainstream school, that they wanted to get together with other teens with hearing loss. Most of these kids were the only ones at their schools who were deaf, and for some it was their only social life. As the club grew, so did the variety of people who joined. We all easily understood each other and would often talk for hours, well into the morning on weekends. Getting together like this helped us hone our social skills and gave us a chance to experience normal teenage social life. In this setting, the subconscious strain or worry of communicating with verbal intelligibility, listening, and lipreading was left behind. Years later, some of us would even find life partners within the group.

A Cathartic Period

My high school years began with two life-changing events. The first was in June of 1985 when one of my best friends, Surekha, died in the tragic Air India Flight 182 crash, the result of a terrorist bomb exploding aboard the plane mid-flight. I will always remember Surekha as one of the most patient friends I ever had on the telephone, never intimidated by the fact I usually had a family member on the other line interpreting for me. Surekha's death was very traumatic. It taught me that life is short.

That was also the summer I landed a leading role in *Crazy Moon*. This gave me the opportunity to be away from home for an extended period for the first time . . . in another city. I learned sign language for my role and continued taking ASL classes throughout high school. My parents were very supportive that I chose to do this and felt that learning another language was extremely important. My brothers had become proficient in French, but I eventually had to drop it because I couldn't lipread when it became more conversational. Ironically, I ended up taking Latin instead.

Because of these two events, occurring so close together, I felt I had grown considerably and had finally figured out more or less what I wanted out of life. I adopted a "seize the day" approach: I wanted to be involved in the arts.

My first high school, North Toronto CI, was academically rigorous and formally structured. The main objective of the school was to get the students into university, and therefore no special subjects were offered outside the traditional academic curriculum. Even the students entertained conformity. When the school bell rang in the morning, everyone looked like they had walked out of the same clothing store. Being the only student with hearing loss there, I realized very much how different I was.

My itinerant teacher from junior high recommended I attend Northern Secondary School instead of North Toronto CI because it had a fabulous arts program and reputedly showed more awareness toward students who were deaf. I was a stubborn teenager, however, and wanted to go where my friends were. It took me a couple of years to realize that Northern was better suited to my needs.

Northern had a program for gifted students and a department for students who are deaf or hard of hearing. Life was much easier and more fluid there. I felt the teachers had a better understanding of my hearing loss and were more accommodating. I decided to have individualized itinerant hearing support since I had to choose either to be mainstreamed with support services or be enrolled in the deaf and hard of hearing department full time. Some of the students who were deaf felt that I was being aloof, since I wasn't attending their classes. That was when I began to realize I might never completely belong in either the "hearing" world or the deaf world. It took me a long time simply to embrace having a dual identity as an "in-betweener."

When *Crazy Moon* was released in theaters in 1986, I had a taste of being a bit of a celebrity at school, although the attention became somewhat nerve-wracking. I would rush home at the end of each day to tune out everyone by watching "The Young and the Restless."

I didn't like to hang around after school since it was hard to keep up with conversations, and I was too exhausted from spending the day concentrating on my lessons as well as lipreading. For the first time that year, I used a notetaker, who provided notes on the infamous smelly and gooey carbon paper. Denise, my itinerant teacher during those years, helped develop my confidence. I became more assertive thanks to her.

University Life

After graduating from high school, I attended York University in Toronto, receiving scholarship aid from the university and the Alexander Graham Bell Association for the Deaf and Hard of Hearing. I majored in art history and studio arts, with additional studies in the humanities. For the first time, I had full access to a complete education. I had a full-time paid notetaker and two sign-language interpreters for each class. More important, I was able to get a taste of what it was like to be a full participant rather than just an observer.

To help support the high cost of being in the Fine Arts program at York — supplies and books were quite expensive! — I worked part time on weekends as a relief counselor in a group home for people who are deaf with multiple disabilities.

In 1991, halfway through my stay at York, I went to New Zealand to play the role of Mabel Hubbard Bell (Alexander Graham Bell's student who later became his love interest and wife) in "The Sound and the Silence," a made-for-television miniseries. My performance as Mabel garnered a Gemini Award nomination (the Canadian equivalent of the American Emmy). I was thrilled and very proud to be involved in this film, which also meant a lot to me personally. We have come so far since Alexander Graham Bell first planted the seeds of the technological harvest we enjoy today in hearing remediation.

As a university student, my acting career took off. I was recruited by several agencies and landed guest roles on various television series being filmed in Toronto. I was often on set and thus required a longer period of time to finish my studies. I graduated in 1994 with a bachelor of fine arts honors degree.

Life as an Artist

Shortly after graduating, I went to live in Paris with Lisa for a few months to develop my skills as a painter. I met a number of people there while learning Langue de Signe Francais and discovered where American Sign Language originated. I got a taste of the rich history behind Deaf Culture. Upon returning to Canada, I went through a phase where I wanted to immerse myself in Deaf Culture and wondered why growing up I wasn't exposed to its stories and history, even as a mainstreamed person who was orally deaf.

Back home, I began to exhibit my paintings, which at that time were adorned with bright vivid colors. A fellow painter described my work as being in the high octaves of sound and wondered whether I painted that way to compensate for my deafness. Who knows?

I didn't like working for one company, nor did I like the traditional 9-to-5 workday. Painting commissions, acting, and contracts with art galleries and art departments for film and television allowed me to embrace what can best be described as a nonlinear career. I set up my own company and have worked in animation, art direction for film and video, and have developed workshops. I also worked as the arts and entertainment editor for the magazine *Deaf Canada Today*. In New York, I worked in a school for the deaf and also painted and sold my artwork. Today, I continue to exhibit my work, sell my paintings, and do portrait commissions in Toronto and New York. In addition, I have helped to spearhead an art and sign studio program which integrates budding young artists who are either hearing or deaf.

In 1997, I met my future husband Jonathan at the Juno awards, Canada's equivalent of the American Grammies. He was intrigued by the fact that someone who was deaf would be interested in such an event. We corresponded by e-mail for a few months before we started dating.

Jonathan is very outgoing, energetic, and has a *joie de vivre* approach to life! He has never treated my deafness as a hindrance. In fact, every time I have asked for assistance, such as having him to make a phone call when I became impatient with the telephone relay service, he questioned why I couldn't do it myself or find an alternative solution. He always insisted I focus on my strengths and independence.

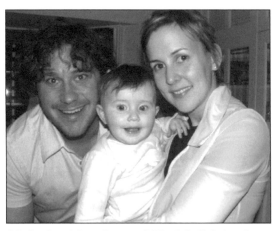

My husband Jonathan and I had Stella's hearing tested just three days after she was born.

Jonathan will never fully comprehend the intensity of what I went through growing up, and I unintentionally placed high expectations on him in the beginning. Fortunately, through joint therapy with a wonderful counselor (herself a child of parents who are deaf), we were able to overcome minor hurdles and our relationship is stronger than ever. Living with a person from a different culture or with different abilities requires a lot more patience and time to fully understand the way the other may see life.

Auditory Therapy . . . Again

By the age of 10, I was excited because I didn't have to attend weekly sessions with Miss Crawford anymore. When I turned 12, I needed braces and intended to use that as a tool for getting out of therapy for good. My ploy worked — and it wasn't until a few years later, when I turned 16, that I took more interest in my speech development and decided that I wanted to return to therapy. I approached the Learning to Listen Foundation where I was welcomed into an already full schedule. Maintaining the Auditory-Verbal skills on which I had worked so hard for many years became important again. I began to realize that learning to speak and listen was like learning an instrument. Without practice, you become rusty.

I periodically continued to see Warren at LTLF throughout high school. I shared with him deaf-related art and film projects, and he inquired at one point, "Why only do *deaf* projects?" Why not projects of interest in general?" I took this advice and before long was flourishing in tackling subjects close to my heart.

A Big Decision

It was during my time at university that I began to notice my hearing aids weren't working well, so I went shopping for new ones. Those I obtained were only mildly better and, by the time I graduated, I had begun to rely more and more on interpreters. I thought maybe my hearing was declining, so I underwent additional hearing tests. It turned out that my left-hand corner hearing loss was becoming progressively worse. I was hearing less and lipreading was becoming more and more tiring.

I was well aware of cochlear implant technology, but I was uncomfortable with it. It seemed rather invasive, and I couldn't imagine how much better it would be than the hearing aids.

A few years later, I finally decided to seriously consider the implant. I could no longer hear the phone ringing right beside me, and I sometimes forgot whether I was wearing hearing aids since they no longer helped me. My residual hearing was disappearing.

When I made the decision to go for it, everyone in my family seemed worried and wanted to make sure that this was what I wanted. I must admit I was surprised at first that my family didn't seem too eager for me to push ahead. All they wanted, however, was for me to be happy and at peace with my decision. My family was ready to support me all the way.

I told only a few friends that I was going for the surgery. I wanted to make sure it worked and that I had made the right decision entirely on my own. The reactions were mixed. One friend who is deaf was upset and said, "You are beautiful the way you are. Why are you allowing yourself to be fixed?" Another friend who is hard of hearing was surprised but very supportive. She said she would do the same thing if her hearing declined.

When I found I was a candidate for the implant, I continued to waiver back and forth about whether it was the right thing to do. I knew the decision would be absolutely final when I was on the operating table looking up at the bright lights. Of course, I know for sure now that it was the right decision. If I hadn't gone through with it, I wouldn't be able to melt at every gurgle and coo Stella makes, the way I do now.

With the cochlear implant, I returned to using the services of LTLF to learn to listen. Interestingly, I was with the therapist when I heard a bird chirp for the first time. I was shocked to learn it didn't sound "sing-song sweet" like I had imagined all my life. It sounded instead like unpleasant squawking.

As I write this, it has been two years since I received my implant. I can hear the birds chirping, the sound of my dog lapping water, and I recognize my parents' voices on the telephone. It was a heartwarming gift to be able to converse with them long distance while I was living in New York, where I got my first cell phone. I never dreamed that one day I would be strutting down the streets of Manhattan talking away with a phone pressed to my ear.

Conclusion

My father was once on a panel of parents of teenagers who were deaf. When asked what he would do differently if he could turn back time, he replied that the only thing he would change would be to grant my wish of having a pet dog. Growing up, I had begged him week after week, month after month, for a puppy — to no avail. Nevertheless, I was surprised his answer had nothing to do with my hearing loss. (I am happy to say that today I do have a dog, a much-loved 8-year-old Boxer named Nina, who also acts as my hearing dog.)

Each child, each parent, and each family is unique. To have a child is a gift, and hearing loss can be treated as a bonus rather than a disability. There are wonderful experiences to be enjoyed and important life lessons to be learned, and through this journey you and your child will meet many marvelous people.

As I look back at what I have written in this chapter, I am reminded of the African proverb, "It takes a village to raise a child." Now that I have a daughter of my own, I can see clearly that it does take a village to raise a child. My mother and father were my primary caregivers and opened their arms to many people — family, friends, neighbors, educators, and professionals — as I grew. All of these people influenced me and helped me become the person I am.

There is no right or wrong way to raise a child. By giving unconditional love, teaching your child the virtues of life, and guiding him or her with the necessary tools so he or she can grow into an independent, functional individual, you are doing your job.

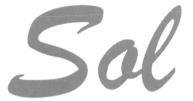

CHAPTER 7

Sol Fried

My road in life has been a difficult one, with one challenge after another. Yet, despite the many years of laughter, sorrow, love, frustration, music, art, education, and friendship, I have matured and my dreams have slowly started to come true.

Looking back, it seems as though everything that has happened to me occurred just yesterday. I remember counting the days anxiously for five years before my Bar Mitzvah. Now, however, it's hard to believe that was nine years ago. And in those nine long years, which now seem as though they were just one, there was my time at Upper Canada College (UCC) in Toronto.

Illness Strikes

I was born at 7:16 on the snowy evening of January 12, 1983, weighing 8 pounds-8 ounces. It was a happy day for my loving parents, a family doctor and a nurse. The same was true for my smiling, redheaded siblings: Golda, Ari, and Shawn. Golda was the oldest, 10 years my senior; Ari was seven years older and Shawn five. Much to my dismay, I am still the baby of the family!

For the first couple of years of my life, I was an active, happy boy with a bubbling personality. I also was cute, I'm told, with fat, rosy cheeks. I was loved and enjoyed by all my uncles and aunts, grandparents, cousins, friends, and our German shepherd dogs. My favorite movie back then was *Superman;* in fact, it was the only movie I would watch.

However, while watching *Superman* one morning when I was 2, I suddenly shouted "Mommy!" and collapsed. I lay stiffly — my eyes, full of emptiness, staring off into space.

Within 20 minutes, I was at the local hospital, where the on-call pediatrician performed a spinal tap. The fluid was so horribly thick that the doctors had to suction it out with a syringe. Blood samples were taken and an intravenous drip started. It was a most frightening time for my mother and father.

I remained in that hospital for three weeks. My parents were told that I had contracted hemophilus influenza Type B meningitis. I was treated with high

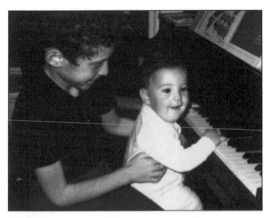

My brother Ari holds me as we have fun at the piano. I was an active, happy boy until age 2, when I contracted Type B meningitis, which caused my hearing loss.

doses of ampicillin, chloramphenicol, and hydrocortisone. I also endured numerous tests, including CT scans, an EEG, an ECG, extensive blood work, and further spinal taps. After 10 days of treatment in the hospital, I slowly began to show signs of improvement.

I arrived home a rather different child. My weight had dropped from 35 to 20 pounds. I had regressed to bottle-feeding and even needed to wear diapers again. I could not walk, sit, or even hold my head up without support. My left side was completely paralyzed. My left elbow and right knee were so swollen that they could not be straightened. There was only pain and frustration. The saddest thing was that my family and friends no longer saw me smile or laugh.

For the next few months, my mother put me through exercises every hour to strengthen my muscles. I continued to be bottle-fed and would scream if a stranger came into view. Eventually my family was able to put me into a stroller and take me for long walks. It was during these strolls, when my mother would point out beautiful creatures such as bluebirds or squirrels, that she noticed my complete lack of response.

Fears Confirmed

By the end of August, a specialist confirmed my family's fear: I could not hear. I was labeled severely to profoundly deaf. My right ear gave no response to the hearing tests, and with my left ear I was able to detect sound only to 2000 Hz before it dropped off to nothing at all. In an attempt to shrink the swelling of the brain still further, my doctor gave me a 2-week dose of cortisone. Irreversible nerve damage had already occurred, however. It was at that point that the doctor kindly informed my parents about schools for the deaf and trained teachers at hospitals in Toronto. My parents were not sure what to do.

I was fitted with two hearing aids which I constantly pulled out. To my parents' dismay, hearing aids were not as easy to fit as glasses. I also couldn't understand what I heard with the hearing aids. My parents found out about Auditory-Verbal therapy and decided they wanted me to learn to listen and talk. They were determined that I should grow up and live, as much as possible, like any other child; they certainly wanted me to attend a regular school.

Fortunately, my parents found a therapist who had the courage, patience, and sense of discipline to have me as his pupil. For an hour each week, my mother and I would see the therapist. We played games and learned to recognize environmental noises and the sounds of speech that so troubled my brain. I remember how much I loved the therapist's collection of toy animals.

After our sessions, I would practice with my mother throughout the day and night, since I could sleep for only about 4 hours at a time — if I slept at all! The Auditory-Verbal therapy and a lack of sleep continued for many years, and as I grew older I learned to listen and converse in sentences.

Finding Myself at an Early Age

My siblings went to a parochial school so they could learn Hebrew and about Judaism. I went there, too, in my preschool years. I loved playing with the other kids in the playground, especially the girls. Before I started kindergarten, however, the principal told my parents that I would have to leave because I was deaf, even though he knew I had the potential to be a successful student since my brothers and sisters were so great in class.

Luckily, my parents found a very small public school that had only one class per grade and no more than 150 students from kindergarten to sixth grade. It was a friendly school where everybody knew everyone else. I remained there for eight happy years and matured into a fine young student, if I don't mind saying so myself.

Despite therapy and my loving family, school itself was not enough for me. I wanted to become the kind of student who was able to carve out a deeper and broader education for himself later in life. Throughout my elementary school years — initially to my frustration, later to my joy — a formidable itinerant teacher would pull me out of class for special support and training for several hours each week. At first, I did not appreciate this opportunity and felt angry. I did not want to be different from my peers, and did not want to leave the classroom. Sadly, some of the other boys made fun of me, and that hurt.

I had heard that a child is supposed to know more than 2,000 words when he or she enters first grade, but I knew only 326. My mother wrote down words in big bold, colorful letters on cardboard cutouts and we would play word games with them. The pile of cutouts slowly grew, and so did my vocabulary.

I didn't learn the multiplication tables until late in third grade, nor did I start to enjoy reading until then. Instead, I cherished learning to play the recorder, going on field trips — especially the zoo — and the great games of dodge ball with my energetic classmates.

An Enduring Friendship

Attending such a small school made it easy to know everyone, and I did make friends (well, mostly acquaintances). A person needs only one true friend — a best friend — in order to be content. And I did make a special friend. As it happened, that special friend's little brother was also hearing impaired and would soon enroll at the same school. He, therefore, had an understanding of what I was going through in life.

My fellow students enjoyed recess and lunch break the most. For the girls, it was a time to chat away; for the boys, it was the chance to drain our energy by running on the fields, playing football, soccer, handball, baseball, and basketball. I would join in, even though I wasn't a good thrower, subject to deep pain because of juvenile arthritis. Fortunately, as I approached my final year of elementary school, my body strengthened and so did my mind.

I found out that my friend wanted to apply to a private school for junior high. Since we were such great buddies, I wanted to go wherever he went. So I applied to the same private school. My aunt found out about this and told my mother, "Sol might as well apply to Upper Canada College, where my son is!" And so I put my name in there, too.

I had never written a real test before and was understandably afraid that I wouldn't pass the entrance exam to this private school. My special itinerant teacher and I worked on the topic of religion, something not at all related to what my class was studying. Eventually I was ready to write my first real exam, which required me to produce both short and long essays.

I had an interview at the first private school, but it didn't go well — not because I wasn't prepared, but because I felt the reception I received at the school was cold and unsympathetic. As we walked out of the admission office, I told my parents that even if I was accepted, I wouldn't go there.

My first impression of UCC was very different. The campus was enormous, with level green playing fields and huge, old trees. The grounds were dominated by both a preparatory school and an upper school, the latter boasting a magnificent clock tower comparable to London's Big Ben.

The hallways of the prep school were filled with energetic boys in uniform, all of whom constantly seemed to have smiles on their faces. The teachers were smiling, too. Even better, the school had facilities for just about every sport.

At the end of our tour, the interviewer surprised us by asking my parents to wait in the lounge while he spoke with me privately in his office. That didn't frighten me, for I was bubbling with enthusiasm about the school. We kept my parents waiting for more than half an hour, neither of us looking at our watches for fear of being rude.

I left UCC that day in love with a school I never thought would accept me. I knew, however, that I had not done at all well on the French section of the entrance exam. All I did was sign my name.

Succeeding at a Higher Level

Upper Canada College has been the longest, and also the best, chapter of my life to date. I am a graduate now — an "Old Boy," as we are called. My eyes moisten as I look back.

I was a fortunate boy, excited by dressing up each morning in a smart uniform. I was going to a school filled with countless other boys my age, and in some way it was a wonderland. I still remember my first day when I couldn't figure out how to open my locker, finally asking for help from my housemaster — a lovely woman and wonderful, supportive teacher.

The world, though, is not always perfect, even in a young child's imagination. In my first year, some of my classmates made fun of me. They bothered and hurt me because I was deaf, with very visible wires running from my waist to my ears. But my heart was determined to show them all that I deserved either to be their friend or to be left alone. I am thankful that my housemaster, the headmaster, and some teachers provided me with great support, encouragment, and praise for my achievements.

The bothersome boys gradually left me alone and started to appreciate me, and they even gave me an occasional smile. As the weeks went by, I tried out, made the cuts, and joined the prep volleyball, track and field, and swim teams. I also became the lead flautist in music class, even though I occasionally lost time when the whole class was playing. I was better at solos.

I had as many as nine teachers for nine different courses. I finally learned some French, and was able to maintain the class average in that subject. I loved science and looked after a pet rabbit in the lab, and I learned about Canadian history. But my favorite subject was English because I studied wonderful plays, poems, and stories — especially Shakespeare. I just love his works. I even memorized Macbeth's entire dagger scene.

Among my new friends and many acquaintances at the UCC prep school, I was fortunate to find one true friend whose father also happens to be hearing impaired. His name is Jonathan, a redhead like me. He was a rather shy boy when we first met, but that has changed, and his parents are grateful for the influence I've had in building his self-confidence. Jonathan and I enjoyed our classes together and talked during lunch hour while gulping down our chocolate milk. He didn't pursue the same sports I did, but we remained friends, supporting each other through good times and bad.

I graduated from the prep school with honors and was pleasantly surprised to receive an award for citizenship, which is presented to a student in eighth grade for his contributions to school life. My mother cried when the entire audience stood as I shook the hand of my headmaster and the Honorable Lincoln Alexander, governor-general of Ontario. Life, I must admit, was very grand at that moment.

Moving on to high school was scary, however. I wasn't sure what to expect exactly, only that I knew it was going to get tougher academically. I was sad to leave so many familiar faces at the prep school: the teachers, staff, and nurses, all wonderful people whom I had come to love during my two brief years there.

> I would not have survived school without my FM system, though it didn't work very well. I often spent recess photocopying friends' notes.

The upper school at UCC — with its imposing clock tower — was big. I was grateful to have Jonathan as my friend. Even though his courses were slightly different from mine, I was still able to spend quality time with him every day.

Since elementary school, I have used an FM system, which helps me hear my teachers more efficiently. I would not have been able to survive without it, even though it didn't always work very well. In the upper school, I relied a lot on my classmates to share their notes with me, which was especially important for my history and science classes. During recess, I would photocopy their notes in the library.

English class was difficult in terms of note-taking. Too many people talked in English class, as students were encouraged to share their opinions of a literary text with each other and the teacher. In that situation, the FM system was not much use. The teacher was not the only person talking, but he was the only one who wore the transmitter. Therefore, for my English studies I relied on reading all of the assigned works on my own and creating my own responses to what I had read without knowing my classmates' opinions. I rarely spoke up in class for fear my opinion had already been expressed. To state the same idea again would have been embarrassing.

My first term at the upper school was just as much fun as it was academically demanding. I discontinued my music lessons since solo performances were no longer possible. But I remained involved in athletic competition, continuing my pursuits in volleyball and swimming. Instead of track and field, however, I became involved in the amazing sport of rowing.

Indoor training for rowing is both mentally and physically demanding. One's heart burns after an ergometer test. One doesn't want to breathe or blink or even stand, for it is all too painful. But once on the water, my soul is at peace. There is no feeling like braving the waves of Lake Ontario at 5:45 each morning from late March until the end of October. It was my chance to be a Greek hero — one of the Argonauts — to accompany Odysseus or to row like Ben Hur.

I love the water. To me, it is a therapy in itself. It relaxes me; it calms me down. Swimming allows me to fly like Superman, and rowing is like magically hovering between air and water, being in neither one nor the other, but reveling in both.

Although most of my fellow rowers tended to be zombies in those predawn hours, my soul felt lightened. The water would remain very calm, almost glassy, broken occasionally by swans, ducks, or Canada geese. As the wind blew at my back and the sun rose slowly over the still faint horizon, its color almost pink, almost orange, I felt thrilled.

I was unable to hear when I rowed or swam with my teammates. In swimming, a teammate would stand at the pool's edge and tap my leg when the starting gun sounded, and in rowing, the coxswain and I developed an exclusive sign language. It was our secret tongue, but very much common sense. For instance, if he wanted more power, especially near the end of a hectic 2-kilometer race, he would put both fists into the air and show off his muscles. Despite our efforts, we never won a race, but we always had fun and I felt we won in spirit.

A Life-Changing Experience

On Valentine's Day morning in 1998, when I was halfway through ninth grade — my first year at UCC's upper school, in the middle of swimming season and indoor training for rowing — I awoke and, as usual, showered, dressed, and put on my hearing aids. Only I couldn't hear anything. I changed the batteries but still couldn't hear. I switched the hearing aids to the opposite ears, yet still nothing. I had become completely deaf

It terrified me. My mind trembled. I needed to hear.

My worst fear at that moment was that I would have to leave UCC because I could no longer hear. Thankfully, the school was very supportive. The administrators and my teachers found various ways to make my days more relaxed and efficient.

When I went to classes such as English or history, I faced the risk of falling asleep — such is the curse of deafness, when you have no choice but to sit still, doing nothing and hearing nothing. It was agreed that I was to do all my work in the school library and report to my teachers on an individual basis for assignments and tests. The exceptions were science and math classes, where most of the teaching was done either at the chalkboard or visually through lab work.

Once again, I visited various hospitals for tests. I underwent both an MRI and a CT scan, and was relieved to learn that I didn't have a brain tumor. To this day, the doctors aren't quite sure why I again had lost my hearing. Perhaps it was stress. Perhaps it was a long-term side effect of the childhood meningitis. Nevertheless, I needed to hear. I had always relied on my hearing aids, and since I couldn't lipread well, those who wanted to communicate with me now mostly had to write things down on a notepad.

I realized that if I wanted to hear again, I had only one option: a cochlear implant. Once, when I was still wearing hearing aids, my therapist asked me if I would consider having an implant. My immediate answer was "No!" — I didn't want to become some cyborg from Star Trek. With $4^1/_2$ years of high school left, however, I was in a desperate situation.

I endured still more tests, including a unique balance test and, worst of all, a crude auditory nerve stimulator test. My lipreading skills rapidly progressed to the point where people no longer needed to write things down, but I still decided, with the blessing of my family, to have the implant. The date for the operation was June 2, 1998, immediately following the Canadian Schoolboy Rowing Championship regatta at Saint Catharines, Ontario (my first experience with such intense competition). I shall always remember that regatta, with gratitude to my teammates, their parents, and the coaching staff.

> I realized that if I wanted to hear, I had to get a cochlear implant. I didn't want one, but with $4^1/_2$ years of school left, I was desperate.

Three-and-a-half months after that terrible Valentine's Day morning, I received a Nucleus 24[®] cochlear implant in my right ear — the ear in which I had always been unable to hear anything at all. I decided to save my left ear in case my hearing should come back one day, or until medical technology progressed still further. One must always maintain hope!

That first night after the surgery was a painful time that my mother and I will always remember. I could barely sleep; I awoke every 15 minutes to ask, "Is it morning yet?" only to see my mother shake her head, "No." For pain, the doctor only gave me Tylenol 3[®], but I certainly could have used some morphine.

The next morning, I went home, very happy to be leaving the hospital since I feel home is the best place to heal. One of my siblings sent me an electronic get-well card that showed a wolf howling under a full moon. It read: "How's Frankenstein doing?"

The doctors wouldn't let me do any physical activity that summer, especially after also having all four of my wisdom teeth removed a month later (to get all the surgery over with). Because of my love of rowing, I decided to build a recreational rowing scull more than 22 feet long. This model, known as "The Kingfisher," was designed by an American named Graeme King; I found out about it in the magazine *Wooden Boat*. My neighbor, an elderly man who would become like a loving grandfather to me, acted as my mentor on this project. He was a good role model, having built canoes, grandmother clocks, and even his own summer cottage.

Another reason I wanted to build this special boat was that the coaches had refused to allow me to row solo. They feared for my safety, even though they knew I had plenty of common sense, was one of the most experienced rowers on the team, and would use my eyes wisely on the water. My boat project kept me busy throughout the summer and actually wasn't completed until the following year, since school "got in the way." Rowing the boat I built with my own hands is one of my greatest pleasures. I have named her Silent Success, which also will be the title of my autobiography when I write it.

But, getting back to my cochlear implant: A little more than a month after my operation, I went back to the hospital for my first "tune-up" (also known as "Hook-up Day"). The doctor first took out my staples, creating a tingling sensation with each extraction. Then I was left with an audiologist and two researchers in a small room. I was fitted with a body processor to wear on my belt and a wire to pass under my shirt; this connected magnetically to the scalp behind my right ear.

I wrote the following letter on my first day back to hearing:

July 7, 1998

Day 1: "Hook-up Jour"
 The CI sounds are horrible. I cannot hear on the phone, understand the radio. I cannot listen to MOZART or any music at all. The noise is like I'm a midget and everything else is a giant! Voices are horrible, too. All speech sounds as if it has been chopped up into syllables, and there always seems to be an echo. Also, some people, like my mother, have a soft voice; thus it's harder for me to comprehend her when she speaks — I can barely hear her at all!

 I was on the verge of crying but would not permit myself in front of the audiologist.

 I started therapy today during dinner with Mom. Here are the exercises for this week:

PERCEPTION PATTERNS
Name Recognition:
Sol
Ema (Mom)
Abba (Dad)
Shawn
Ari
Golda
Sheba (Dog)

Six Sound Test (6): a(r) oo ee sh s m

Phrase Patterns:
Happy Birthday (4 syllables)

Sol (1 syllable)
Bye Bye (2 syllables)
I want to go home (5 syllables)

Change the set configuration:
No
Maybe
I'm hungry
Want to go to the movies

Single Words:
Bus
Ice Cream
Elephant
Hippopotamus
Dandelion

I went over these with Mom in the following steps:

First, I'd read the words or sounds using my own voice.

Second, I'd listen to Mom as she reads the words while reading her lips at the same time.

Third, I turn away from Mom's lips and she says the words behind me and I tell her what she is saying.

Fourth, Mom tells me if I'm correct or not by giving me the thumbs up or down.

Fifth, Mom repeats the above, but each time in a different order.

Sixth, the above is repeated more than ten times for each of the four sections, or until I become too tired.

Seventh, we both SMILE.

When one already knows a word, it's easier, but still hard despite the fact that one of only four words is being said. Since it sounds like a different word. I'll say what I hear, not what is actually being said! But I must be corrected; I must learn that the word I hear is not 'dish' but 'fish'!

The therapy is very tiring and DOES frustrate me! The sounds produced by the CI are 100% different from what I heard with the hearing aid. When a soldier listens to his walkie-talkie in combat and there is a lot of static and interference . . . that's basically what everything sounds like to me. I have to rely on my memory of the sounds I heard with the hearing aid.

Each time I turn on a tap to or flush the toilet, it sounds like I'm standing underneath Niagara Falls!

My brain has to adjust to these new noises. How long it will take for me to hear on the phone and be able to listen to music is unknown, since everyone's brain is different. I'm hoping that it will be SOON!

I'll try to keep writing about my experiences with these alien sounds on Planet Earth.

Once again, I had therapy with the same therapist I'd had as a child. It was frustrating, but thankfully this time I had a decent vocabulary and could read, too. The therapist pushed me, and once I even cried during our session. I hadn't cried in a long time; in fact, not since my beloved grandfather had passed away three years earlier, just when I had successfully finished my first year at UCC. The word I could not distinguish was a simple one: church. My therapist consoled me, saying that it was good to cry. He wanted me to cry, and indeed I did feel better afterward.

Three months later, I could talk on the phone, although I still needed repetition from the person I spoke with most of the time. Patience was required. It took 6 months before I became used to the implant.

Meanwhile, I continued to go to the hospital every once in awhile for another "tune-up." I felt like a piano, just as fragile, just as musical. I graduated from auditory therapy once again, six months after that first "tune-up" day. I continued my studies, my horseback riding, and my involvement with sports at UCC. I also did some drawing and painting, and I discovered a love for the theater, especially performing on stage. It was in the theater, in fact, that I met my first sweetheart.

Dating: A Whole New World

While I was learning the waltz for a play that was written, produced, and directed by students, my dancing partner teased me about a girl in her school who would be just perfect for me. Having attended an all-boys school for six years, I was more than ready for some female companionship.

I didn't meet Melanie until after the second performance. She first saw me at my best, in a tuxedo on the dance floor. Upon meeting her, I took her hand and said, "We will be perfect for each other, as you can hear for me and I will see for you." She has trouble seeing with one of her eyes and, yes, she was the sweetest and most beautiful person I had seen in a long time. She was just 5 feet tall, with long dark hair and sparkling hazel eyes. The saying that "Good things come in small packages" is certainly true for her.

The following evening, after the final performance, I went to her home and we talked until the small hours of the morning. From then on, we held hands, went for long walks in the park, and visited art galleries, Toronto's wonderful zoo, and the Casa Loma castle. We dined out and went swimming. We even went to our schools' dance parties. Melanie came to watch me row competitively, even though she knew that I couldn't hear her cheering me on.

Our relationship lasted a year, until she left Toronto to go to university. Things were never 100% perfect: we had different religions, and I was too much of a country person for such a big city girl. But she will always be a part of me, and remembered with love.

Expanding My Horizons in Scotland

I always knew that I wanted to go to the University of Guelph near Toronto, with the goal of becoming a veterinarian. I occasionally visited there on my own and even went so far as to meet with the associate dean of the Ontario Veterinary College. By his reaction, I knew I was on the right path in terms of both academic achievement and life experience. Gaining admission to the program of my dreams, however, was going to be challenging.

When I was in 11th grade, an admissions officer from the University of Glasgow in Scotland visited UCC early in the school year to recruit applicants. The UCC university placement adviser and I were the only ones to show up for the meeting. This was a perfect situation for me since I perform better communicating one-on-one. Knowing that Glasgow had a veterinary school, I told the officer of my interest and about my experiences. He responded cautiously, expressing concern that success in the program wasn't likely because of my disability. Although he wasn't encouraging, he did promise to be in touch after he had informed the veterinary school about me. I didn't hear from him again until a year later when UCC received a letter saying that he would be returning to the school accompanied by the veterinary school's admissions officer. Apparently she wanted to meet me for herself.

At the meeting this time, there were two other students; however, despite the extra company, I managed to impress the admissions officer. (I especially amused her by saying that the only connection I had with Scotland was my red hair.) I learned afterward that the officer found it hard to believe she had met and talked with a person who was deaf. We kept in touch by e-mail, and I eventually arranged, with my parents' blessing, to be interviewed by the Glasgow admissions committee the following summer.

I traveled to Scotland on my own and arrived in Glasgow on August 26, 2001. I did not understand a word the taxi driver said in his thick Glaswegian accent. But he somehow managed to get me to my accommodations at a local bed and breakfast. I surprised the admissions officer by calling her on her mobile phone to let her know that I had arrived safely. That was the first time I had actually "spoken" with her since we met at UCC nearly a year before — and we were talking on the phone. I spent the afternoon exploring the university. It was beautiful. The following day I explored the small town of Stirling, with its ancient castle and huge Victorian monument to Sir William Wallace (of *Braveheart* fame). It, too, was beautiful. At 5 the next morning, I went rowing on the River Clyde along with 12 swans — surely an auspicious omen. Then it was off to the capital city of Edinburgh to visit its lofty castle and the Royal Mile.

> I learned afterward that the admissions officer found it hard to believe she had met and talked with a person who was deaf.

Three days after I arrived, I finally had a chance to meet with five members of the veterinary school admissions committee: three women and two men. It was the first time I had faced so many adults at once. The interview, which lasted slightly more than an hour, involved many questions. One of the committee members purposely tested my hearing by covering his mouth while speaking to find out whether I needed to rely on lipreading to understand what he was saying. Thanks to my training in Auditory-Verbal therapy, I was able to pass these tests, even when allowing for the Scottish accents.

That evening, I received welcome news. Once again, I quickly put my thoughts and feelings into writing with a letter to my family and friends:

Scotland is of utmost beauty, and my soul will be greatly content to study there. The land is filled with endless lush greenery, trees of great height, and vast mountains of valiant strength.

The University of Glasgow is built of mighty stones and iron gates. Its ancient buildings are a sight to see. The veterinary school itself is located in a "secret garden" along a river. And, aye, I did indeed row on the city's River Clyde the morning prior to my interview at five o'clock, alongside twelve swans that had flown down from heaven.

I must make haste. I shall now reveal some merry news that may indeed bring a joyful tear to your faces.

I . . . have now been offered a place to study in the Faculty of Veterinary Medicine of the University of Glasgow commencing in October of 2002.

This offer is conditional upon my achieving a final average of no less than eighty-five percent, a task that, fear not, I will accomplish with determination and love for my studies.

I shall be the first of my kind, or from Upper Canada College, to study veterinary medicine at Glasgow, and perhaps in all of the United Kingdom.

I thank you all for being there for me throughout my life. Without you, I would not be who I am today.

I spent my final year at UCC focusing entirely on my studies, engaging in no extracurricular activities except to complete the Duke of Edinburgh's Gold Award program and competing for my seventh consecutive season on the school's varsity swim team. It was a good final year, though at times very stressful. My dream was within reach. I worked hard, earned a final average of 90%, and graduated on May 24, 2002. At the Leaving Ceremony, I was honored with an award, this time for perseverance in the face of adversity. I am very thankful to UCC and shall miss the supportive community there. But there is a time for everything, and the time had come for me to move on.

Exposure to the Working World

Just as my deafness has not prevented me from completing my secondary education, the same can be said for working effectively with veterinarians, technicians, and clients. In fact, my work experience has made me stronger, more determined, and appreciative of others. It also has helped me focus on my goals. The veterinarians I have assisted have given me the strongest encouragement to pursue my career choice. I have been very fortunate to find wonderful people to work with and learn from.

Because I was determined to gain as much experience as possible while pursuing my dream, I spent five years as a student at UCC volunteering at both large and small animal clinics. I observed many procedures, and helped out whenever an extra hand was needed. In the summer of 2000, for instance, I temporarily left my family after my brother's wedding to work at a kibbutz in northern Israel. There, I learned how to farm a dairy herd of more than 750 Holsteins. It was one of the greatest adventures of my life.

When I returned from Israel, I didn't think my experience with cows, horses, cats, and dogs would be enough to convince any veterinary admissions committee of my eligibility, so I decided to try something unusual for a person my age — laboratory research at hospitals in Toronto. Fortunately my family had contacts within the Toronto medical community that permitted me the chance to do research work. I took that chance and proved to my fellow workers and supervisors to be a diligent and efficient research assistant who could work successfully alongside others. I was invited to return the following summer.

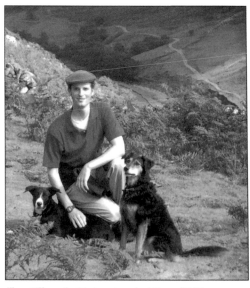

Collegiate Struggles

I decided to pursue my studies at Glasgow instead of the University of Guelph because I would be able to enter directly

I'm still undecided as to what I would like to do. Do I follow my lifelong dream to be a veterinarian, or do I have a future as a Mountie?

into the professional degree program from high school. I had waited nearly two decades to do that and didn't wish to delay any longer than absolutely necessary.

My two years there gave me a wonderful opportunity to study abroad and to experience Scotland's rich culture and history. The Glasgow veterinary school is among the oldest and most reputable in Great Britain. I am very proud to have been its first student who was deaf or hard of hearing, as well as the youngest ever to enroll from North America.

It is thrilling to know that Glasgow is the same school where the renowned James Herriot was trained before starting his veterinary practice in Yorkshire. Am I destined to follow in his footsteps?

I made four journeys to live in the land of Herriot with a wonderful English family and their dogs. Each Easter holiday, I helped a farming family with the lambing of their 350 ewes. It was very peaceful living in the clean country air of Yorkshire surrounded by lush green valleys and dales, with the wild heather growing on the distant moors. Two families there have become my "English" home . . . my friends for life.

All the same, I had no immediate family in Scotland and often wished to return home to Canada. I had chosen a most difficult path. Indeed, my life would have been easier to have studied in North America, where professors speak with an easily understood accent and support services during lectures (such as live captioning) are available. Since those support services were not available for a foreign student in Britain, I had to rely on the kindness of other students to obtain copies of their lecture notes.

Lectures continued to be tiring for me, which meant I often had to go to the library and study from the textbooks. There were many lectures in which I actually fell asleep, despite sitting in the front of the class. I just wasn't able to comprehend the lecturer's voice even with the aid of an FM system. The lights were often turned off so students could screen projections with greater ease — thus, I was prevented from lipreading. I was at a great disadvantage.

After enduring two full years of studies and examinations, I was informed that I had not passed second year. I felt angry, frustrated, humiliated . . . and alone. So, I packed up my belongings to return home to Canada. I had had enough. Even though I was on the path toward fulfilling my dream, I realized that I was studying in the wrong environment and it was time for a change.

It had been nine months since I had last been home and I fought back tears on the flight to Toronto. I was happy to be returning to Canada, however, with its wonderful cultural diversity. Still, although my family was happy I had returned, I lacked a personal sense of peace.

Rethinking my Options

My first week home, I went to an information session for the Toronto Police Service. I sat at the front and introduced myself to the two recruiting constables giving the presentation. I shook their hands, said my name, and asked them if they would wear the FM system (after explaining what it was). Although I didn't show it, I was upset when they refused and informed me that my deafness would be a liability. [Obviously, they had not heard of FBI agent Sue Thomson, who reads lips and knows sign language.] Nevertheless, I sat in the front and heard everything. I was able to see one of their medical officers the next day. I informed him that I had just returned from studying in Scotland and that I wanted to help people, with a long-term goal of working with the mounted and/or canine units — thus, still working with animals. I handed the medical officer my audiological report showing that I could hear within normal ranges with the cochlear implant in my right ear. The medical officer noticed that for the left ear the audiologist had written DNT, which means "Did Not Test." He asked about my left ear and I explained that I was saving it for future technology or medical advancement and that the implant was only in my right ear. The doctor was not sure if the hearing requirements for constable duties needed to be bilateral, but he said he would look into it and then let me know where things stood. I thought to myself, "Well, I can always have the implant in my left ear as well." I shook his hand, stared deep into his penetrating eyes, and left. He didn't keep his word, however. I never heard from him again.

Two days later, I attended an information session in Toronto on becoming a Mountie with the Royal Canadian Mounted Police (RCMP). This time there were three constables involved and I received an entirely different welcome. The constables were more than happy to wear the FM system while they talked, the session was informative, and I could see that the constables were excited and enthusiastic about their careers.

I received an e-mail from a corporal in the RCMP to indicate that if I can hear with the cochlear implant, becoming an officer shouldn't be a problem for me. After reviewing its sample tests on the Internet, I know I can do well on the RCMP examinations.

Someone once told me that the RCMP "needs good people like me as its representatives." My mother, though, believes I will be sent to a "boot camp" somewhere on the other side of the country. Personally, I think it would be like going to overnight camp in the great Canadian wilderness. It would be fun.

However, although I would be proud to wear the RCMP's bright red jacket and black pants, with riding boots and wide-brim hats, I have asked myself if I am ready to change courses and forget my lifelong dream of being a veterinarian.

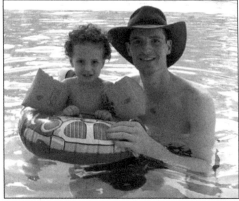

I have discussed all my options with family and friends, but ultimately the decision is mine. To leave as many doors open as possible, I wrote to the University of Glasgow to see if they would be willing to let me return as a student. Officials there gave me permission to do so in September of 2005, but I remain undecided.

If I do return, I know that I need to seek more help, and I would need to visit my family in Canada whenever I got the chance. I will no longer think of the veterinary program as a five-year course, for I am young and as long as I succeed in becoming a veterinary surgeon one day, does it truly matter how old I am when I graduate? Returning to Glasgow to become a veterinarian would be a "means to an end." But is it worth the price?

I remind myself each day to be patient, have heart, persevere, love life, look at the positive aspect of every situation, give others a smile, and smell the roses.

As I write this, I have begun working on my B.A. in English at York University in Toronto. I was somewhat scared to start fresh at a Canadian university; however, I also am excited, for I know I will meet new people and make new friends. Plus, it gives me the chance to study other interesting subjects such as literature and psychology — reacquainting myself with the Arts. I intend to rediscover a whole world of knowledge out there besides veterinary medicine.

Challenges Ahead

I have a challenging road yet to travel, and plenty of adventures to come. I know many more days of both joy and sorrow await me. I remind myself each day to be patient, have heart, persevere, love life, look at the positive aspect of every situation, give others a smile, and smell the roses. I will always remember that I could not have achieved what I have so far without the endless support, advice, and love of my family and friends.

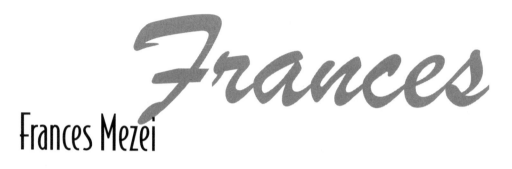

CHAPTER 8

Frances Mezei

My journey with hearing and listening has been a gift. The successes and challenges I have faced throughout my life have enriched me — and the members of my family — in many ways. My family, in fact, has been encouraged to break barriers and explore new possibilities in the field of hearing loss. Today, I lead a natural, productive life and am a functioning member of the community, mainly because my family provided me with the necessary communication skills to thrive in society and to feel positive about myself.

My hearing loss was an important impetus to my destiny and my spiritual journey. It has helped me connect with who I really am. I have learned the freedom of the human spirit, which has helped me communicate with anyone.

Diagnosis and the Early Years

I was born in December of 1957 . . . at a time when technology and education were very different than they are today. When I was 2, a doctor in Toronto confirmed what my parents had suspected earlier: that I had a profound hearing loss. This was a different diagnosis from the ones I had received from the other doctors who had examined me. My problem, they had concluded, was that I was just stubborn. They also told my parents that they couldn't test a child's hearing before the age of 2, a scenario that unfortunately was all too common in those days.

The doctor in Toronto who examined me wrote:

> "I feel her delayed speech is the result of perceptive or nerve type deafness of unknown etiology. . . . Before formal education is available for her, a great deal can be done at home by the use of lip reading and amplification. . . .As an introduction to amplification, an experimental hearing aid has been loaned. Mrs. Mezei was disappointed and upset by my findings — this was especially true when she understood that because the nerve elements of the ear are affected, nothing can be done to restore hearing."

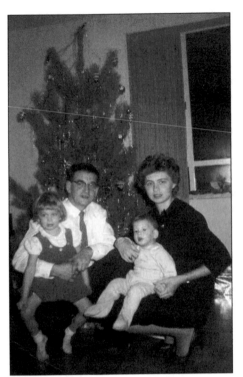

My mother attended the doctor's appointment by herself. My father acknowledged later that he had made a mistake not to be at that meeting with her, a decision he said he deeply regrets. To this day, he tries to be present for all important doctors' appointments for the family.

It was a terrible shock for my parents to hear the news of my hearing loss, almost as if I had died, or at least that their dreams for me had died. They went through the grieving process with confusion, anger, despair, and frustration — disadvantaged especially by a lack of expert information on deafness. There were no parent sharing groups, and they were unaware at first that even with my deafness I had the potential to learn to communicate. My parents were worried that I would never learn to speak and cope with life.

The certainty of the diagnosis did provide some relief, however. They could finally understand why I had not reacted in certain ways and they could begin to educate themselves on what needed to be done to help me. The doctor's suggestions to teach me to lipread and use hearing aids was a good starting point as my family began a lifelong process of education and hard work.

Despite their initial shock, my parents immediately started to concentrate on what could be done rather than dwell on the misfortune they faced.

Despite their initial shock, my parents immediately started to concentrate on what could be done rather than dwell on the misfortune they faced. My mother never let the thought of "what could have been" enter her mind, which made it easier for all of us to focus on the reality of the present.

The first family battle came with my refusal to wear hearing aids. At first, I resisted violently. The only time I would accept them was before going to sleep and only if I could climb into my brother's crib or be taken for a walk in my stroller. Overall, it took 6 long months of conflict and compromise to finally accept and cherish my aids. I have worn them ever since.

My speech and language education began in earnest. My mother, with her indomitable spirit, determination, and patience, proceeded down that winding road to provide many years of daily lessons to teach me to identify sounds, make words, and then link them into sentences. Her task was not easy, since I would often beg to play with my friends instead. Every day, however, my mother insisted that we complete our lesson before doing anything else. Since my mother and I were both stubborn, and each of us wanted our own way, one of us would eventually start crying. My father and my brother would often bet on whether the lesson would be "a wet one or a dry one."

My brother, who was two years younger, willingly served as my interpreter in those early years when people couldn't understand what I was saying. The clarity of my speech varied; my parents understood me more than others did, but my brother understood me best. Once, when I was 5 years old, I was screaming and crying and no one could understand why I was upset. It was my brother who said, "She wants a cookie." My parents gave me a cookie and immediately I stopped the tantrum and became happy again.

The doctor in Toronto who had diagnosed me was influential in the field of hearing loss and remained an influence for my parents both as a guide and a coach. Shortly after my diagnosis, he referred us to the correspondence course of the John Tracy Clinic in Los Angeles (since nothing was available in Toronto in those days). For two years, my mother exchanged letters with experts at the clinic and received guidance and support on how to train me to lipread and, through extensive use of visual objects, to talk. I progressed quickly, using a combination of lipreading and "hearing" to develop an understanding of many new words. My mother kept a list of words that I knew, and within six months I had a vocabulary of 400 words. I approached anything new with great resistance — I had an independent mind and a determined character, and I was not always ready to follow my mother's instructions. This did not last, however. She would concentrate on the things that I liked and casually check whether I was ready to work on the things I had previously resisted.

From 1960 to 1963, my mother wrote letters to Roundabout, a support group for parents of children with hearing loss from different parts of the United States and Canada. I recently received a precious gift from my father. He gave me these letters to help me write my story for this book. I was finally able to learn about how my dear mother assisted and nurtured me throughout the years — in her own words! This wonderful gift filled an important gap about my early upbringing. Due to a serious illness, my mother passed away in 1977, when I was 19, but I share the following comments from those letters. They moved me deeply.

> My brother served as my interpreter in those early years when people couldn't understand my speech. The clarity of my speech varied.

Francie loves to be told about names of various objects; she is very interested when things are explained and usually keeps asking for more. She loves picture books and actually goes to the library with us and borrows books for herself. Right now discipline is really the bigger problem than lessons. She is always eager to learn; however, she has not learned to listen to us. Firmness on our part usually works wonders; she improves and starts behaving beautifully. To be firm and consistent with discipline is not easy, as you all probably know, and yet it is essential in my case. Francie's behaviour has improved tremendously. If she does get upset about something, a simple explanation calms her down. The important thing is how to get some things across to her, which has become easier, since her understanding of language is always progressing. I find that patience on our part in explaining things to her is very important; it makes her accept certain situations without too much upset, and it also makes her feel very important. We talk to her about everything that is happening about future events, and she usually nods her head very knowingly or adds her own comments.

My father recalls the day I grasped the word *later.* There were countless occasions when my parents couldn't explain that the treat or the trip was coming, only not now, but later. Suddenly I was able to connect a word with an abstract idea. I finally understood, and it changed our lives.

In a letter from August of 1964, when I was 6, my mother wrote the following:

> *Francie definitely knows now that she can not hear as well as other people. She asked me once, "Can Michael (her brother) hear?" I said, "Yes, Michael can hear." Then she asked me later during the day whether I could hear. I said "Yes" and she said about herself "I can't hear." To her, this seemed just an ordinary conversation, as if she was talking about different colors of eyes. Lately, she often says "I can hear it" after adjusting her aids.*

My parents enrolled me at the Metropolitan Toronto School for the Deaf when I was 3½. When the doctor responsible for recommending my educational placement tested my hearing, he was impressed with my progress and wondered why my parents wanted to send me to a school where I would acquire some of the "mannerisms of children who were deaf." My parents felt, though, that my language skills hadn't developed sufficiently and that I needed special help. But, at that time, there were no other local support facilities or clinics to assist us.

At the Metropolitan Toronto School for the Deaf, however, my progress slowed dramatically and I even had to relearn vocabulary that I had previously acquired at home. In my three years there, my parents constantly asked themselves whether I was being challenged enough. Some of the teachers felt I wasn't ready for the change to a "hard-of-hearing class," and the principal gave my parents the discouraging prognosis that I was a "deaf child" and would always have to go to schools for the deaf. My parents faced a major dilemma: either leave me in that school or find a regular school for me somewhere else.

Fortunately, in 1964, we were introduced to Louise Crawford, a pioneer in Auditory-Verbal therapy who worked in Toronto. I was privileged to be one of her first "students" and worked steadily with her for four years. We had lessons once a week in order to develop good speech, a good command of language and, especially, more refined listening skills to complement my lipreading skills. I admired her firmness and steadfastness in striving to pioneer new ways to educate children to listen and speak. This was her vocation and her deepest passion. I commend her vision, integrity, and devotion in bringing opportunities and freedom to the lives of many children, including myself. She encouraged my parents to follow their heart's desire to integrate me into a regular school, but she warned them that they wouldn't receive much support by making this decision.

An excerpt in my mother's diary explicitly describes her feelings about this:

> *I am frightened by what we are trying to do and yet I am determined to go through with it. The book "Our Deaf Children" by Freddy Bloom started me in this direction and Louise Crawford convinced me that we are doing the right thing with Francie.*

As I was about to enter first grade — after spending three years at the Metropolitan Toronto School for the Deaf — my parents made a courageous move and transferred me to a private school: Bayview Glen.

Before making this life-changing move to an integrated setup, my brother and I spent four weeks at a day camp run by Bayview Glen to check my readiness for a group of "hearing" children. I was very happy at camp and my language and speech improved considerably. As my mother cited in her diary:

> *Francie is attending day camp with hearing children. She likes it very much. She does have problems when there is singing or story telling. She tells me they sing "fast, fast, fast," but I have a few of the songs written out for her and she keeps reading the camp songs enthusiastically at home, and she thinks she is singing. It really is very cute!*

When I was 7, I transferred from Bayview Glen and became one of the first children with hearing loss to be placed in a regular class in the Toronto public school system. To this day, I shudder wondering what would have happened if my parents hadn't made that move. Their decision enhanced all my future choices and options. I will be forever grateful to them for crossing what was an unimaginable and insurmountable barrier in those days.

It was an exciting time for us. My vocabulary started to grow by leaps and bounds, new concepts became familiar to me, and my voice intonation improved. I passed first grade with good results and continued on to second grade. Second grade was an even better experience since I understood much more of what went on in class. My teacher also helped tremendously by tutoring me privately every Saturday morning.

Involved Parents

In 1961, the first seed for the organization that would become known as VOICE for Hearing Impaired Children (VOICE) was sown when my father joined the principal of the Metropolitan Toronto School for the Deaf and several other individuals to form the Metro Toronto Association for Hearing Handicapped Children (MTAHHC). In the early days, many of the MTAHHC meetings included guest speakers, plus there was a parent sharing group and a library with valuable resources. In addition, there were several fundraising events. A great deal of work was done by mothers such as Ann Griffith, Joan Beattie, and my mother Annie.

In 1965, my mother presented a talk on the importance of reading, which was well received by her fellow MTAHHC parents. She made several excellent suggestions, such as:

> *Reading is the only means by which children who are deaf can overcome their isolation. It has often been said that people who are deaf are characterized by a certain immaturity — this is natural since they miss so much of what is being said. Unless they learn to enjoy reading and acquire an understanding of the world through reading, they might remain very childish and naive indeed. Children usually imitate their*

parents and become interested in the things their parents enjoy. For this reason, I feel parents of children who are deaf must first develop an interest in books and reading themselves. . . . I realized in our own family that our children hardly ever saw me read. . . . I am trying to change now. . . . Since Francie was three, I think she has been going to the library with us and selecting her own books. At first, I was too eager for her to get books with easy factual material — no fantasy stories for her, who has so many concrete words to learn. I feel now that I was mistaken. Francie loves stories of giants, dragons, fairies, and stories with a plot. They are far better because they are more imaginative and interesting. . . . At one point, I was terribly pleased when Francie started crying when a sad story was read to her. I knew she really understood and experienced it. When it first happened, she couldn't understand why her eyes filled with tears, and I explained to her that it was because the story was sad.

While my mother worked hard to develop my communication skills, my father performed an important role in the new organization. He often served on the MTAHHC executive board and even served as president at one point. Along with other parents, he lobbied strenuously on our behalf. He wrote petitions to the Canadian government to obtain audiologists for the city, to encourage mainstreaming in the public school system, and so forth. In 1967, Toronto finally obtained the services of its first audiologist. Until then, hearing testing had been very rudimentary.

My father also prepared briefs and brochures, and contacted the media in order to obtain itinerant teachers for students with hearing loss in the public schools. In 1969, the school system employed its first itinerant teacher, who worked at that time with seven children with hearing loss. The service expanded quickly, and today itinerant teachers are available in nearly all school districts in Ontario. I began receiving itinerant assistance when I was in third grade, while attending the public school in my neighborhood (a service that lasted through the end of high school). Each itinerant teacher, I'm happy to say, had a different influence on me — each invaluable.

My mother and father were the first parents from Toronto to attend an Alexander Graham Bell Association meeting in the United States. They learned first hand about the latest developments in oral education and about auditory training. As a result of my parents' trip, Toronto quickly became a hotspot of Auditory-Verbal activity. Leaders in the field frequently came to the city to speak and consult.

It was in 1965 that VOICE was officially established. The organization dedicated itself to the principle that every child, regardless of the degree of hearing loss, be given an opportunity to develop spoken language and listening skills that would ensure they could function effectively in the hearing world.

My father became the chairman of VOICE in 1977. In the spring of 1978, he went with several parents and the coordinator of the Toronto school system's itinerant program to North York General Hospital with a plan to establish a clinic that would enable children to learn to listen and talk. Louise Crawford's program at the Hospital for Sick Children was fully booked at that time and another therapist was urgently needed. The head of the ENT department at North York agreed to set up an auditory training clinic. After a slow start, several parents (including my father) were able to recruit Warren Estabrooks from the Toronto District School Board to serve as the clinic's lead therapist. Warren became the director of the Auditory Learning Centre of the Learning to Listen Foundation and the rest is history. I was privileged to work with Warren for a few months before he was obliged to turn his full attention to working with the newly diagnosed babies, toddlers, preschoolers, and school-age children at the clinic.

We are so fortunate today that the power and hard work of all those parents helped turn the dream of an auditory clinic for children with hearing loss into reality.

Struggling to Keep Pace

I spent third grade at our neighborhood public school, but the road to academic success was not always smooth. I constantly struggled to catch up with my school work. My language skills were always limited and I often missed what was taking place in the classroom. My mother, fortunately, was always on her toes. She would meet with the teachers regularly to find out what topics we would be discussing in the classroom so we could prepare ahead of time at home. She found it a constant struggle and worry.

I, too, found elementary school very trying. Because the other kids were unable to accept my "difference," they made fun of me — to the point I felt I had no future. A few kids teased me, laughed at me, and called me names. That really hurt. Years later, when I was in high school, I vividly remember planning to confront the boy who had been the ringleader in taunting me in elementary school. In my final year, I approached him in the hallway one day and told him what he had done. He apologized and I got all of the angst I felt off my chest. Perhaps these trials fueled my resolve in pursuing my goals and helped me acquire coping skills to protect myself.

When I finished elementary school, my teachers were very concerned about my readiness for junior high since I had done poorly on the English examination. The principal, in fact, requested that a psychologist come to the school to administer tests to see whether I should move on to junior high. The psychologist's tests showed that I was "bright, alert, determined and capable and should not be held back." What a life-saver that was! I found out later that many other students in that elementary school also did poorly on the English test. I had been singled out because of my deafness. My parents always felt that if you waited until you were ready to do something, you would never be ready. So, I made my way to junior high school as scheduled. To the relief and delight of my parents, the principal of my school also had a daughter who was deaf, so he was understanding and helpful. I was the first person in Toronto to have access to an FM system. My parents had gotten it from a Bell Canada engineer who worked with Daniel Ling at the Montreal Oral School, and I was able to use it in school

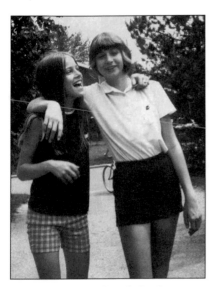

One of my closest friends in the neighborhood was Monique (left). Today, we say that we "made each other's childhood."

as an experiment. I proudly carried around the big, black professional briefcase with my new device, which consisted of a microphone plugged into a small FM transmitter and a big radio connected to a "mini-loop" attached to my hearing aids. I was a hit with some of the students because whenever the teacher left the room, they asked me to turn on the radio. After a year of use, however, the novelty of the FM system wore off. It became an inconvenience to carry such a bulky briefcase. Today, I use an FM system frequently, but to my delight it is much smaller.

In high school, I did fairly well. I was an average student and, like others, I found that some subjects were easier than others. I recall one tough social science teacher who always challenged his students to expand their limits. He gave us an interesting assignment to write an essay detailing the means of surviving alone on a desert island for one year. I reread my story recently and was rather amused. It is 21 pages long.

The subjects I enjoyed most were art, playing the clarinet, and workshop, where I made sculptures out of wood and metal.

Special Friends

For 15 years, my family lived in a modern bungalow in a friendly, quiet, and peaceful neighborhood in Toronto. My mother wrote in her diary about our friends from that neighborhood.

> *Francie spends most of her day playing with her brother, Michael, and her friends. There are many children her age living in the houses around us, which is a wonderful thing for her. She likes company and the children seem to enjoy her, too. Some are very cute in trying to talk to her, very slowly and exaggerating each word! I am very careful in not correcting them too much, thus making them self-conscious. I hope they will eventually learn by following my example to speak naturally. Some still motion to her, and I try to discourage this. On the whole, however, I am very pleased that she gets along so well with hearing children.*

It was a different scenario at school, where I found it difficult to make friends. I was unsure how to communicate with children, and I had to work very hard academically. Every day after school, I was anxious to come home so I could play and relax with my family and my two best friends. Although I had few friends who were sensitive to my hearing needs at school, I was fortunate to have had two close friends in the neighborhood. Today, my friend Monique and I tell each other that we "made each other's childhood." I would sleep over at her house and go on trips with her family, and vice versa. This friendship was a true joy in my life.

I also took ballet for a few years and enjoyed it. As my mother once wrote in her diary:

> Francie did well in her ballet group this year. One of the most pleasing things was to hear the teacher telling me that she forgets that Francie is in class and that she doesn't have to give her any special attention.

Tennis, which I learned to play at a young age, and bridge were highlights of my childhood. My family often played these games together.

I am told by other family members that my inability to speak well and to understand everything had a great effect on the family. For example, I often dominated the dinner table conversation and would interrupt others in a loud voice because I didn't realize they were talking. I was also a main topic of conversation with my parents' friends since they found my progress interesting. As I got older, this kind of attention decreased greatly and my mother's long illness became a more frequent topic.

Always an Inspiration

When I was 10, my mother was diagnosed with a terminal brain tumor. She struggled with her illness and had three operations. After each operation, she managed periods of good, productive activity, including five years on the first occasion. Watching her deal with this, especially during the last three years of her life, was very painful. She had an amazing strength, and every time I visited her at the hospital, she would smile and continue to show me deep love. I watched her suffer tremendous pain, lose her balance and fall, lose her hair, her memory, even her bodily functions. People tell me that her greatest legacy was giving me the unique gift of speech, which ironically she would lose later during her illness.

It frustrated my mother and worried her greatly that she could no longer give me lessons. A few close friends came to my house each week to fill in for her, and for seven years before she died I received valuable weekly lessons from Dorothy Scott, a private teacher whose main focus was developing language and listening skills. Dorothy became a good friend of my mother and always gave her constructive suggestions. Her high standards and firmness fueled my desire to be successful.

My mother passed away when I was 19. The rest of the family rallied to help during this difficult time. My grandparents, aunts, uncles, and cousins were important people in our family. My brother and I had many joyous experiences with our grandparents, sleeping over at their house on weekends, going out to restaurants, and even occasionally traveling with them. It was a special bond. Interestingly, my grandfather never believed that I would speak or cope at all well with life. He always felt sorry for me. My parents generally ignored his worried remarks about me. However, it was my grandfather, a dermatologist, who referred my family to the doctor who diagnosed my deafness.

My parents tried to make life inside and outside our home as normal, balanced, and carefree as possible, which was especially challenging when my mother was ill. However, I have many wonderful memories of trips as a family . . . to Europe and Israel, across Canada in our camper trailer, to Scandinavia, to the

East Coast of Canada and Prince Edward Island, to Expo '67 in Montreal, to Cape Cod, and to Michigan on a fishing trip. During our travels, my parents always talked to me and helped me to name things. We labeled everything. We also enjoyed going to operas, plays, movies, and special events. Fortunately, I have always been curious about everything. My father once told me he was amazed that even when I didn't follow or understand a play or show, I always found something interesting about it or obtained some pleasure from it.

Becoming Self-Reliant

I was very shy and unsure how to relate to others in high school. I was overwhelmed by the way people spoke, and I did not always feel comfortable with my deafness. I would often escape to the school's washroom where, in front of the mirror, I tried to imitate the high level of adult talking. I became obsessed with the question, "What do people talk about?" But I didn't really know what I had missed until years later.

In high school, I became anxious to use behind-the-ear hearing aids. I had always worn Y-cord body aids, and until high school I was never bothered by them, from a cosmetic point of view. Now I didn't want to be seen as different. I asked my parents about this and we went to see an audiologist in Massachusetts. He prescribed a new pair of BTE aids that I loved wearing. They made me feel more comfortable in my surroundings.

It fell upon my father to teach me self-reliance. I remember frustrating times when I wanted my father to help me understand the language of the school textbooks. I wanted help for 2–3 hours a day, but my father rationed me to only 1 hour of assistance. I often felt panic and frustration. Eventually his "limited assistance" helped me become more responsible and independent with my studies. By 11th grade, I could do most of the work on my own. The marks I received averaged between 69% and 72% for each year of high school. In my final year — Ontario schools went to Grade 13 back then — I received a pleasing 74% average, even though that was also the period when my mother died. I missed a month of school while she was in a coma, but thankfully my father continued to provide firm and wise guidance. He believed I had the ability to complete the school work independently.

I didn't associate much with a peer group in high school, nor did I date. At times, however, I did go out with my brother's friends to parties and other social activities. I'm not sure how my brother felt about having his sister follow him, but I always felt welcomed by his friends, which was a blessing. I also recall frequently rushing home after school to be with my mother.

After high school, I attended York University in Toronto for three years, receiving my B.A. in psychology. My original goal was to study art, my favorite subject, but I don't regret majoring in psychology. To cope better with the lectures, I asked fellow students to take notes and gave them sheets of carbon paper to use at each class. I sat in the front and would always explain to the professor about my hearing loss, but I was still too self-conscious to use the FM system. I always thought it was too much bother. Today, many universities and colleges have centers for students with disabilities, and I wonder how different my experience would have been if I had had such special support.

I developed wonderful friendships at the university, both male and female. We often got together to talk or go to dances and parties, I also went cross-country skiing with a male friend almost weekly for a few years. One winter, I went to a movie with a friend when there happened to be a strong flu bug going around. While we were standing in line to buy tickets, I suddenly felt very weak, my knees started to wobble, and I fainted. My friend panicked and called for an ambulance. When the ambulance arrived, the attendants noticed that my speech was not clear and asked whether I was drunk or taking drugs. "No, she is just deaf," he explained.

While at York, I was asked by a Toronto radio station to write a poem about what it felt like to be deaf. The following is my poem, which was heard across the airwaves throughout Ontario.

> *I wonder how it would feel*
> *To hear the birds singing,*
> *To hear the raindrops falling,*
> *To hear the people whispering,*
> *And most of all*
> *To hear the children playing.*

Exposure to academic mainstreaming, despite its challenges, provided me with many skills. I think the earlier one is exposed, the easier it is. It is also essential to have the care, love, and assistance of parents when dealing with the myriad complexities of the school system. It is the parents' job to nourish and prepare their children for progress, provide them with skills, and nurture self-esteem and confidence so they may have the proper head start to participate fully in society.

A Blended Family

A year after my mother passed away, my father married Kathy, who also had a child who was deaf, 10-year-old Patrick. My family moved in with Kathy's family in a historic heritage house (circa 1855) in the Toronto suburbs, what was once a farm. Suddenly we were introduced to many new people and it took time to adjust. Since Kathy had three children of her own, our family expanded to seven people.

At first, there was tension. Each member came into the new family with his or her own preconceptions and expectations of how parents and family life should be. Many accommodations needed to be made, such as the types of food we ate, how the house was kept, and how to relate to a new set of family members (e.g., step-grandparents, aunts, etc.). We also had to get used to different cultural backgrounds. Kathy's family consisted of seven Canadian generations; mine was European and Jewish. One big success was that each person, including the youngest child, Patrick, had to cook once a week. We posted a calendar on the fridge and each of us had to sign up for a cooking night.

It was challenging in the beginning and I experienced much confusion and anger, among many other conflicting emotions. Gradually, however, I was able to take on the role of student again, after spending a long period as "housewife" for my brother and father. I enjoyed the new freedom.

All of the adjustments we made helped the family become flexible and open-minded to new ways of functioning. I feel we have done extremely well because of great efforts on everyone's part. Plus, we have learned to respect each other's individual characteristics.

My relationship with Patrick was the most interesting. My father told me that at first it was strenuous. Because we were both immature, neither of us was sensitive or understanding of the other regarding our communication needs. For example, we sat next to each other at the dinner table, and whenever we talked, we did not face each other, which caused comprehension problems. Eventually, we changed our seating arrangements so that we faced each other across the table, which was much better. Today, I am happy to say, we both have understanding and respect for each other.

Among my more cherished memories are the summer vacations we took to the cottage on Lake Couchiching, north of Toronto, where Kathy and her mother spent their summers as children. These vacations gave us an extended opportunity to enjoy each other's company. Our large family dinners were special, with many children of all ages, and also public occasions and performances. I found it very relaxing when Kathy would interpret orally for me. Fortunately, we still enjoy these moments today.

The 'Saturday Night Club'

In my adolescence, I became aware of the social isolation and loneliness that many teenagers with hearing loss feel when they attend a regular school. As a young adult, my friend Sarah Jane and I, then 22, organized a support group called the "Saturday Night Club," which consisted of about 35 teenagers with hearing loss. We met once a month at my family's home, went to movies, had parties, went skiing or skating, and basically enjoyed as many social activities as possible. The initiative greatly exceeded our expectations, since whenever we got together there were gales of laughter, constant talking, and beaming faces — everyone felt at home! We understood each other and could be ourselves. We relaxed and developed many long-term friendships. Although these teens were younger than me, it was the first time I felt my heart open up and my frustrations melt.

A few years later, I was also a member of the steering committee for the youth section of "A Sound Beginning," a conference organized in 1985 by the Canadian Hearing Society (CHS) and the Alexander Graham Bell Association for the Deaf. The challenge was to coordinate a national youth conference for Canadians with hearing loss to celebrate the International Year of Youth. About 100 youngsters from across the country attended this successful conference in Toronto, expressing sentiments similar to what we had experienced with the Saturday Night Club.

I shared my experiences coping with hearing loss during numerous talks, including one titled "Don't Be Afraid to Be Different," which I delivered at the 1983 A.G. Bell Association convention in front of about 1,000 delegates. Looking back, I am very grateful to have been involved in these activities.

Embarking on a Career

I held various jobs after graduating from York University, such as a recreational counselor for the Ontario Housing Corporation and public relations worker for the Office of Sport for the Physically Disabled. I also worked for several years in the Ontario Provincial Government as coordinator for an employment program for youth with disabilities. All these jobs were stepping stones for the real job I wanted: teaching communication skills to those who had lost their hearing. My inspiration was a workshop on aural rehabilitation I attended at the 1985 "A Sound Beginning" conference.

In 1987, I called the regional office of the Canadian Hearing Society, using my TDD to make the call. I asked a secretary I knew there whether any jobs were available. She said she had been thinking about me and told me of an opportunity that would allow me, finally, to channel the skills built during my volunteer work into a full-time career. For the next seven-and-a-half years, I worked as an employment and community outreach counselor at the CHS, a position of constant change and growth. Working in a friendly office with 10 other employees was a real pleasure. My work included preparing clients for job searches and linking them with various placement agencies, in addition to helping employers make the workplace accessible. I devoted a great deal of time to organizing support groups for individuals and seniors who were hard of hearing. I also worked as a counselor and taught lipreading and communication classes to individuals who had lost their hearing later in life, and to the elderly. It was a joy to observe how people developed new skills to cope better with their hearing loss.

> I taught lipreading and communication to people who lost their hearing later in life. It was a joy to observe people develop skills to cope with their loss.

My work there culminated in joint authorship with Shirlee Smith of *Lipreading Naturally*, a published guide to lipreading and communication that serves as a practical teaching resource for those working in the field. Among the topics covered in the guide is role-playing, and there are creative "field-tested" exercises that students can use to improve their communication skills in everyday activities such as shopping and traveling.

I also developed a program for women escaping violence, and for three years organized a week-long Elderhostel Program for seniors with hearing loss and their spouses.

Leap of Faith

While working at the Canadian Hearing Society, I searched for new meaning and purpose in my life as my mind buzzed with many unanswered questions. I developed two close friendships with individuals who were Bahá'ís. I asked them many questions about the Bahá'í faith and attended meetings with them, eventually becoming a member in 1989. It changed my life. I shifted the way I perceived and approached my hearing loss. It helped me refocus from dwelling on my physical limitations to the importance of spiritual nurturing and the strength of the soul. It also taught me how to acquire virtue and develop personal talents. I became aware of the importance of expanding my spiritual hearing, and passionately sought the physical and spiritual truths of the concept in order to enhance living. Physical and spiritual hearing are complementary, I discovered.

The following Bahá'í quote had a powerful impact on me:

> *Wherever in the Holy Books they speak of raising the dead, the meaning is that the dead were blessed by eternal life; where it is said that the blind received sight, the signification is that he obtained true perception; where it is said a deaf man received hearing, the meaning is that he acquired spiritual and heavenly hearing.*

Shortly after becoming a Bahá'í, I moved to Puslinch, Ontario, a small town just west of Toronto, where I have lived for the past 14 years. Over time, my small Bahá'í community and I have explored, through consultation, ways to adjust to my hearing needs. At meetings, there is always an empty seat beside me so others can sit on that chair when they read out the prayers, letters, or correspondence. That way, I can read the written words they hold. I wear an FM system, which helps me greatly, and I always make sure there is sufficient lighting. People put up their hands when speaking and face me so I can lipread. From time to time, I need to remind people of these strategies because they do forget. When I become frustrated, I remind myself that it is my job to educate others in communication skills. One person told me that my Bahá'í group has learned how to slow down and really listen to others.

In 1994, I longed for another change. For about 6 months, I had suffered from extreme dizziness and vertigo, which at times incapacitated me. That proved to be another turning point in my life. It was a sign that I needed to begin an inner journey and learn to take better care of myself. I left my job at CHS and began an enjoyable year at Sheridan College in Oakville. I explored my heart's desire to study art and to discover the artistic skills that were buried deep inside me. I took classes in photography, design, painting, drawing, and printmaking. I discovered my ability to paint, using the medium of watercolor, something that I continue today.

During that period, I felt very tired from all the hard work as well as stress in learning to communicate. I was also still grieving the loss of my mother. I realized that I was a child of parents who were survivors of the Holocaust (my father escaped from his hometown in Hungary and was aboard the Exodus '47 boat that attempted to bring Holocaust survivors to Palestine in 1947 despite a British blockade; my mother spent 18 months hiding underground with her parents in Poland). I needed time to allow myself to heal, relax, and acquire new skills to communicate with others. I had to revisit my painful past to cleanse my soul from pain that had persisted under the surface for years. I went through all the stages of grief (anger, negotiation, depression, and acceptance) at different times in my life in order to accept my hearing loss, my mother's death, and many other changes.

I went through cycles of acceptance, of hitting walls, and of crashing down and feeling sorry for myself. Each of these intermittent stages has been important in discovering my potential and my spirituality. It was easy to limit myself by saying "I cannot do this because I am deaf." That restrictive attitude was self-defeating and held me back. However, it took a great deal of effort and persistence to overcome the feelings of ambivalence, fear, and resistance. As I did, I ultimately discovered my desire to be with a larger group of people. I felt my life would expand in unimaginable ways. That was the true path of consciously moving beyond my inner and outer barriers, letting them go, and moving forward.

In 1997, I started an international electronic newsletter called Healing Through Unity, which is published to share thoughts and experiences on how the teachings of the Bahá'í faith are being applied to physical and spiritual health. The current circulation is approximately 2,000 subscribers in more than 110 countries. It is a joy to be able to communicate with people from different cultures and countries. The readers are educating me as well. They let me know that each of us has our own difficulties and struggles to overcome and that we need to assist each other since we all live on one planet as one family. I also have joined with friends to publish *A Journey of Courage: From Physical Disability to Spiritual Ability*, which is a compilation of writings on the Bahá'í perspective of disability.

I continue to be involved in many groups and often wonder how I cope with it all. I still have difficult moments in large groups when a number of people are talking at once. The conversation is sometimes too swift to follow. There are times when I go home feeling tired and frustrated. Time and again, I pick myself up and re-educate the group I'm with. In general, I feel that I gain tremendously from being in groups such as the Town of Oakville's Diversity Working Group and the Guelph Barrier Free Education Committee, as well as attending numerous Bahá'í events. I have been on a number of planning committees for major conferences. I have designed art displays for the Puslinch library, done layout work for the local community newspaper, and organized tennis activities for the Puslinch tennis club. I have a part-time job at Mohawk College in Hamilton, Ontario, and I administer and monitor college exams for students with disabilities. I was honored to receive the 1999 Ontario Community Action Award presented by the Ministry of Citizenship, Culture and Recreation.

> I started the newsletter Healing Through Unity, which shares thoughts on how Bahá'í teachings apply to physical and spiritual health.

I play tennis at the local club, attend fitness classes, and practice yoga. I enjoy traveling and have visited Poland, Israel, and Ukraine (including my mother's hometown), and have journeyed across Canada and the United States. I enjoy being an aunt to my niece Mila and my nephew Alex who give me great joy.

Listening to music is a wonderful pleasure. I want to develop a deeper appreciation for music, so I attend concerts or musicals as often as possible. I also always wanted a guitar, so I went ahead and purchased one. I took weekly lessons for a year, and even though it was difficult, it was a joy to play with the strings. My teacher was very patient and never doubted that I could do it. I also belonged to a drumming group and participated in public performances.

Two Momentous Decisions

On June 11, 2001, I went to a party to celebrate the career of Louise Crawford. That was also the day I decided to get a cochlear implant. The party was attended by many adult implant users who were doing quite well. I felt inspired when Louise told me, "You would do well with an implant." After the party, I conducted intensive Internet research on the subject and went out of my way to ask several implant users how they felt about them.

A few weeks later, I attended the Cochlear Implant Conference in Minneapolis, where I was in awe and overwhelmed as I sat through the presentations on rehabilitation, telephone strategies, appreciation of music, devices, surgery — anything related to cochlear implants. It was as if I had entered a whole new world for individuals with hearing loss, something I had never dreamed was possible in my lifetime. Whenever I asked someone how he or she liked their implant, I was told, "It is a miracle!" However, I needed to understand what the "miracle" meant, so once again I embarked on a journey that changed my life.

I contacted Sunnybrook Hospital in Toronto for an assessment to determine whether I was a candidate. I completed all the tests and became a candidate on January 11, 2002. One of my main concerns, however, was whether I would be able to receive postimplant therapy. I realized that therapy was vital to successfully benefiting from an implant, so I applied to the adult therapy program at the Learning to Listen Foundation's Auditory Learning Centre. Because of their high standards and success with other adult implant users, I felt the therapists there would be the best ones to help me learn to listen again. In my application letter to the Foundation, I wrote,

> *I have reached a plateau in terms of my ability to function in the hearing community, and sense that I need to be released from some of the physical limitations imposed by deafness through the benefits of a cochlear implant and therapy. . . . Some of my responsibilities as a student in therapy will be to work very hard, to be persistent, flexible, determined, have a willingness to let go of my old listening and speech habits, be creative, and have a strong desire to listen to the new sounds.*

I also outlined some of my goals for hearing: a) develop auditory awareness and discrimination; b) develop my listening skills; c) improve my speech; d) speak on the telephone; and e) improve my confidence when communicating with people.

In June of that year, I took another huge step. I decided to adopt a baby girl from China, working with an organization called Children's Bridge, that has assisted approximately 1,600 families in adopting children from China, South Korea, Thailand, and Vietnam. Children's Bridge has a vast array of resources with which to work, such as play groups, e-mail support chat lists, singles support groups, and workshops. It guided me through each step of the adoption process (including all the paperwork) and helped me gain valuable personal insights and understanding by connecting me with other families.

I had to wait until January of 2004, however, to meet my daughter, Diane, from China. Before then, I had to continue planning for my implant surgery.

The Moment of Truth

I had my cochlear implant surgery on April 22, 2003, at age 45. I was unable to have any visitors because of the Sudden Acute Respiratory Syndrome (SARS) outbreak in Toronto at that time. I did, however, feel very happy that I finally received my ESPirit 3G® processor after several delays. I felt great strength from the many prayers I received, and from the support of friends and family members during the surgery and the days immediately following.

To be better prepared for the "hook-up" — and for my own peace of mind — I kept a diary and wrote down several important points during the process. Keeping a diary is vital because it allows you to observe the development and progress of your hearing journey, and it is something I will be able to share with my daughter one day. As I said in one entry:

> It is my understanding that the "static" I hear today will become the beautiful sounds of tomorrow. I will need to take it one day at a time, to experiment and to trust in the process in order to endure this difficult, fascinating and awesome journey to discover the world of cochlear implant sounds. The keys to success for the next six months are patience, persistence, self-discipline and calmness.

My father joined me on my hook-up day, which was June 5 — six weeks after my surgery. First, I was told to listen to the different frequencies. The audiologist turned on each of the electrodes one at a time. I was "feeling" sounds rather than hearing them. I felt pain and had a great deal of discomfort. I also heard lots of awful sounding beeps. I was disappointed; it was not what I had expected. The audiologist was happy, though, saying that the nerves and the implant were in good working condition and that my initial reactions were normal. Then she asked me to listen to a quiet *sh* sound. I had never heard it before, but now I could! I was able to distinguish between *sh* and *ss!* My father broke down in tears when he heard this. "It's a miracle I have dreamed about," he said. We had a good cry, but I felt nervous because I knew that the learning curve before me was a steep one.

I wanted the first words with my implant to be special, so my father read the following from the Bahá'í writings:

> The rewards of life are the virtues and perfections which adorn the reality of man. For example . . . he was deaf and becomes a hearer. . . . Through these rewards he gains spiritual birth and becomes a new creature.

I started to live my childhood again. I had a great time exploring new sounds I had never heard before . . . the clicking of my computer's mouse, the high-pitched twang of a fork hitting a glass, my footsteps, the turn signals of my car, the rattling of keys, my own breathing, the sizzling of oil when cooking food, running water, and so on. I didn't realize that so many things made sounds, and that the world was such a noisy place. My brain started working overtime to identify, discriminate, and comprehend all of these new sounds. I felt overwhelmed and confused, but also excited and curious. I struggled with fatigue the first few months, but that gradually improved over time, just like so many things do.

I enjoyed one memorable surprise about two weeks after my implant was activated. I went out to water my vegetable garden and then walked to the marsh where I heard a lot of noise. There were about 25 birds singing. I had dreamt of hearing birds singing my whole life. I sat outside throughout the summer listening not only to the different bird songs but also the chirping of crickets and the croaking of frogs in the marsh.

Therapy at the Learning to Listen Foundation began soon after that . . . and it was a process filled with excitement, joy, frustration, and growth. The therapist explained that the primary goals of auditory rehabilitation were to promote functional communication skills and fulfill my listening potential. We started with small steps since I needed to relearn everything from scratch.

> I walked to the marsh, where I heard a lot of noise. There were about 25 birds singing. I had dreamt of hearing birds singing my whole life.

At the therapy sessions, we did some basic tasks such as the Ling Six-Sound Test (ah, oo, ee, sh, s, and m); simple questions such as, "When is your birthday?" and "What is your telephone number?"; and counting, colors, and letters of the alphabet. We would start our sessions with me being asked, "Frances, can you hear me?" and "Are you listening?" We also did auditory tracking, which involved following the words in a book by listening to them being read aloud. However, I found this easy from the beginning so we didn't spend much time on that skill.

As therapy progressed, we moved from closed-set tasks made up of a few listed words and sentences to open-set tasks that involved listening to questions such as, "What did you do on the weekend?" and "How many brothers and sisters do you have?" We also listened to compound words such as ice cream and baseball. Some fun (but also difficult) listening exercises involved crossword puzzles, nursery rhymes (to share with my daughter), and descriptions in which the therapist would provide clues about an object and it was up to me to figure out what it was. For example, the therapist said, "I use it in the bathroom to wash my hands" and "It is white." We also started having short conversations, and whenever there were environmental sounds during the sessions I was asked, "Do you hear that?" and "What do you think that sound is?"

I was encouraged to have faith in my hearing and to trust myself rather than just guess. I was taught to take responsibility for occasions when I didn't understand what I heard by asking for a specific word to be spelled. I also learned that I didn't need to understand every word to make sense of a sentence. This helped me to be more relaxed.

At home, I was fortunate to have some excellent helpers. Twice a week, I worked with a retired friend who volunteered to help me for an hour each time. She was motivated and excited about my progress. We did our sessions based on the exercises and techniques taught by the therapist. She taught me a few listening games that I could play with my daughter ("What sound does a cow make?"; "Where is your toe?"). A neighbor of mine also helped from time to time, and I had daily lessons with my father and Kathy at the cottage. Kathy taught me five nursery rhymes that I learned by listening only. She would say one of the lines randomly from the rhyme, and usually I was able to identify the line after a few repetitions. We also did a difficult exercise in which I was required to discriminate between words with different consonants (e.g., pate, bate, gate) and words with different vowels (e.g., tub, tip, tag).

I listened to many children's tapes while following the books. I progressed quickly to a more advanced level and began reading and listening to *Rose in Bloom*, a 300-page book by Louisa May Alcott. I enjoyed it very much; it was natural and entertaining.

I started to practice listening on the telephone with my father and Kathy several times a week. Regular practice seemed to take the edge off my fears. To get started, I prepared a list of common phrases, the names of the members of my family, and short sentences using colors. My father and Kathy would say these to me and I would repeat what they said. Then I put away the list and would tell them what sentence they said by listening alone. We also practiced counting, which worked well. Their feedback consisted of easily distinguishable coded words such as "OK," "No," and "Almost." (I am sure a higher level will develop with lots of practice and time. It is hard work — I get tired after 15 minutes, but I am determined to do it.)

I never realized how deaf I was until my hearing increased with the cochlear implant. For me to hear and be receptive to the sounds that surrounded me, I needed to undo years of adaptation as a primarily visual person. I needed to stop "tuning out" sounds that had previously been just vague, indistinct noise. I needed to really listen. I needed to reduce my visual orientation to the world. Instead of hearing through my eyes, I started to hear through the implant and trust my hearing abilities. My balance in life was upset, and some of my habits and adaptations to deafness were no longer beneficial. I needed to let them go and reorganize my world. The therapist was sensitive to these issues and helped me develop a new sense of orientation, responsibility, and identity.

> I never realized how deaf I was until my hearing increased with the cochlear implant. I needed to stop 'tuning out' sounds that had been just vague noise.

Gradually, I became more alert, listened more attentively, and changed my perspective of myself to a whole person who can hear. I still find it difficult because it is like learning a foreign language, but I have become more relaxed and confident with myself. The world seems a kinder and friendlier place. I enjoy being with people, and communication seems to be easier. I am told I have begun to speak more clearly.

As I write this, I have had my implant for 5 months and there have been times when I have needed to re-evaluate my expectations and goals in order not to be disappointed and frustrated. To find real pleasure in my hearing, I remind myself to live in the moment and allow the process to happen naturally. I strive to move forward in a balanced way and to do all my "listening work" at a comfortable pace. When I become tired, I stop. I know it will take years for my brain to adapt to the new sounds and to make full use of the implant.

At a recent MAPping appointment, my audiologist said it was important for me to develop a tolerance for hearing new sounds, since I had been deaf for many years. She admitted that it is a huge change and adjustment, but nevertheless extremely important. I felt relieved after hearing this. It was my seventh MAPping at which they adjusted the loudness level of the individual electrodes at the different frequencies, matching the settings to my individual needs. Many implant users tell me that it will get better over time. The implant has opened new opportunities and given me much more to look forward to in life. My new hearing caused me to become much more aware of my surroundings.

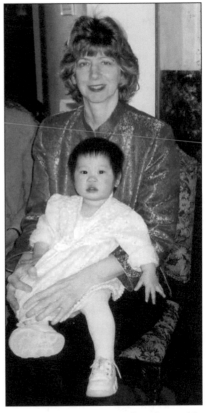

My Child, My Gift, My Blessing

As mentioned above, I decided to adopt a baby girl in June of 2002. In January of 2004, I traveled with my father and 47 other families to China to bring Diane home. My greatest joy is being a parent, and I hope I will continue to follow my parents' example in providing a stable, loving, joyful family environment in which Diane will develop a solid foundation.

It has been exciting to explore the world of sounds and speech with my daughter Diane. We often play music in our home since Diane loves it so much.

My experience with hearing loss has helped me relate to what a child from a different race might feel in terms of fitting in and handling discrimination. I took great pleasure in hearing my daughter's voice for the first time and communicating with her. It has been exciting to explore the world of sounds and speech together. We often play music at our home since Diane loves it. I was excited when I first recognized the song "Old MacDonald Had a Farm" and now I can tell every time it is being played. I will, at times, hear without lipreading certain words that Diane says. She is definitely helping me learn to listen better!

The decision to have a child was my greatest impetus for learning to listen. I have eagerly entered another new phase in my life and am delighted to be able to share it with my little girl. I look forward to continuing the journey for as long as possible.

I understand that being a parent is one of the most complex and important jobs in life. Having a child with a hearing loss makes it even more challenging.

Parents are the child's first and most important educators, and it is essential for them to impart their values and virtues. Parents need to view their child as a whole person and not dwell on the limitations posed by deafness. This holistic approach will enable the child to feel good about himself or herself and develop strengths and virtues. The immersion of the child in a loving, nurturing environment in which listening and talking are the major forms of communication will provide an abundance of lifestyle choices and opportunities. As a single parent with a new child and a new way of listening to the world, I welcome the challenges and trust that life will continue to be bountiful because of them.

I was fortunate to have a solid family foundation and a happy home life. My parents taught me how to listen and how to love, and they nurtured and cared for me in remarkable ways. My father said his biggest concern was that maybe they pushed me too hard to be successful, since there was always the pressure for me to manage well in an integrated school setting. I believe my parents' high standards — and their persistence and patience — were all invaluable in helping me develop the virtues of discipline and responsibility I embrace today. I learned to relax, followed my needs, set priorities, took good care of my health, and eventually learned to listen to and trust my intuition. I now strive not to let my deafness dominate my life or my identity, but rather to use it as a way to learn how to love, share, serve, and show compassion to others.

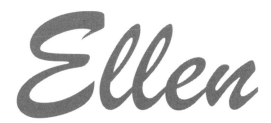

CHAPTER 9

Ellen A. Rhoades

Birth, Infancy, and Guilt

My mother wanted five children. She loved babies. She doted on her first-born, a beautiful and healthy curly-haired little boy. One day, however, her mother-in-law told her that her son wasn't able to hear, which made my mother want to strangle her. She never quite forgave her mother-in-law for saying that, but she was spurred to seek the opinion of an ENT doctor. When my mother learned that her son, then nearly 2 years old, *was* profoundly deaf, it brought her to her knees. My father, just back from serving in the U.S. Army during World War II, gave her moral support and the strength to move forward. Determined that their son would talk one day, my parents began making frequent trips from Long Island to New York City to visit the usual merry-go-round of doctors who might offer them that nonexistent magical "cure."

It was about this time that I was born — my parents' joy somewhat muted by their sorrow at my brother's hearing loss. For the next year and a half, I accompanied my mother and brother on their journeys to the city, going from doctor to doctor. I was the innocent bystander who played quietly by myself while my mother, with her naturally loud and deep-voiced gift of gab, drilled my brother on speech and language through a visually oriented home correspondence course. Given our limited family income, they played endlessly with clay and blocks, my mother learning how to say the same thing in many different ways. She later confessed that she hated these drills because it was so difficult for her to be creative and because she found little or no time for the activities she personally enjoyed.

Regardless, after about a year or so, my mother eventually became suspicious when I, too, did not respond to sound. I certainly wasn't vocalizing. She quickly learned that I was also congenitally deaf — although with an 85 dB bilateral loss, it was not as profound as that of my brother. Her shattered world seemed even bleaker, and she determined not to have any more children. She continued her journey from doctor to doctor, but now it was two children who needed to be treated.

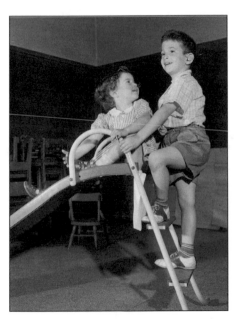

My mother, in search of a miracle cure for our hearing loss, believed a doctor's assistant was a "quack." That assistant was Doreen Pollack, who became a pioneer of the Auditory-Verbal movement.

One day, she took us to a doctor at Columbia Presbyterian Hospital who told her: "Stop shopping around and wasting everyone's time. The most important thing you can do for your children is to give them the best education possible." The doctor had his clinician, a soon-to-be-famous woman named Doreen Pollack, demonstrate that my brother and I still had enough residual hearing that could be used to help us learn to listen. My mother, however, was convinced that this clinician was a quack and wanted nothing to do with her — never mind that Ms. Pollack would soon become a leading pioneer of the Auditory-Verbal movement — but at least the seed of hope for us had been planted.

My mother revealed to me later that during this period of my life I was given no home courses or drills because she had devoted all her energies to teaching my older brother how to talk. After a year or so, she finally acknowledged, "I guess we have neglected Ellen." According to psychological reports written about me, the general picture suggested that my family overindulged me, that I found the role of "baby" too satisfying to give up. I ran roughshod over my brother. He had to let me have what I wanted simply because I was the baby.

In 1947, around my second birthday, my mother learned about an experimental federally funded project taking place in New York. Dr. Ciwa Griffiths was a consultant to the project. Her belief (similar to Doreen Pollack's) was that even young children who were deaf had enough residual hearing that could be tapped with powerful hearing aids, allowing these children to be educated alongside their normal-hearing peers. (This actually was a reverse mainstreaming project whereby children with normal hearing were brought into a language-enriched preschool classroom for children with hearing loss.)

For the project to succeed, parents were expected to participate meaningfully throughout the process. That was acceptable to my parents. My father, in fact, was so intrigued with the project's potential benefits that he moved us from Long Island to the city so we could take part. Thus, I was among the first wave of American preschoolers with hearing loss who would learn spoken language naturally: by hearing it.

I only learned much later that my mother began feeling burdened with tremendous guilt during this period. With no known cases of deafness in our extended families, she took the blame for bearing two children with hearing loss. When she was pregnant with my brother, my father was fighting overseas. She didn't feel it was a good time to have a baby, so she took special pills to induce an abortion. Although the pills didn't work, my mother believed that ingesting them caused our deafness. It wasn't until 50 years later that the science of genetics absolved her of that heavy burden. Our deafness was, in fact, caused by connexin-26, a protein deficiency, but that knowledge really didn't alleviate either of my parents from the deeply hidden abiding sorrow that they carried until their deaths.

Preschool, A-V Learning, and Pity

Although it was rather revolutionary in 1948 for young children who were deaf to use amplification — even if just for a few hours each day — I immediately responded to a hearing aid. As soon as the rather big and clunky body-worn aid was given to me when I was little more than 2, my parents saw that I liked to wear it, that it enabled me to hear quite well, and that I started to vocalize. Despite the fact that most of the professional community at that time did not agree with Dr. Griffiths' notion of early amplification, and even though my parents had trouble affording it, they purchased two body-worn aids: one for me and one for my brother. It made perfect sense to them that with such a powerful hearing aid I should be able to learn to listen and understand what I heard. And so, for the rest of my life, I became a single-sided hearing person, with the aid placed on my left ear.

At the same time, I started attending the language-enriched preschool alongside children with normal hearing. During the first phase of the pilot project, which included learning natural spoken language through normal group play activities, I was the subject of several written reports. Each morning, when my mother dropped me off at class, I would scream and cry when I realized it was time to separate from her. However, I always regain my composure quickly and became my usual cheerful self, losing myself in group activities.

My regular preschool teachers felt that I was highly intelligent. They reported that I was "shy and reserved at first," yet one who was "always a happy, spirited member of the group, who played well with other children." They further wrote that I "possessed a sense of adequacy" in all that I did; that I seemed very much at home in the world and in touch with what was going on. They added that I "easily accepted new people, situations, and routines" largely because of "warmth, friendliness, and interest in people and things." I seem to have taken everything in stride, was able to hold my own in a group, and made definite contributions to the life of the group. I was, they reported, "cooperative, friendly, alert, independent, and self-assured with a wonderful sense of balance and coordination."

In the second phase of the project, my mother accompanied my brother and me to Vassar College in Poughkeepsie, New York, where we, along with a handful of other mothers and children, stayed in a dormitory for a month during the summer. All the mothers participated in daily group discussions and educational meetings while the preschoolers, including their siblings with normal hearing, engaged in a variety of play activities. That month, my mother was finally able to embrace potential normalcy for us as a family.

After the summer, I happily resumed my preschool experiences, again in a class alongside children with normal hearing. The teachers reported that over time, as I warmed up to more of my peers, I did my "own share of directing the activities of preschool playmates." I learned language naturally from just playing with other children. My teachers reported that I had "a healthy curiosity towards new experiences, and a wide range of interests." I was "a merry, cheerful, gay, lively little girl who sometimes bubbled over and was generally relaxed." Everything I did seemed to provide satisfaction, and I shied away from those few activities that might have frustrated me. When I did engage in those activities, however, the frustration usually passed very quickly. As the teachers noted, I "showed little or no anxiety most of the time and seldom was aggressive." They also noted that I "spoke freely, making excellent progress in speech and language, largely due to her excellent use of residual hearing."

My parents quickly came to understand that good amplification and optimal use of residual hearing was our ticket to the "hearing" world. They expected us to listen at all times and, when we didn't, they showed annoyance or anger, depending on the situation. My mother, in particular, was a very proud and forthright woman who was honest to a fault. She didn't like being the center of attention and she disliked pity. In our preschool years, my brother and I each had body-worn hearing aids about 6 inches long and 4 inches wide "You should see them in the subway in New York City," my mother said one time. "When I take my children in the subway, I feel as if I am a freak. I feel I want to try to hide them because everyone looks at them with their hearing aids, and they are so aghast you see all sorts of expressions on their faces. I dread going into the subway with them. I guess the most difficult part of being a mother of children who are deaf is freezing up when other mothers ask questions about them, and pity you and them."

She would often recall the time a minister saw us in the subway and told her that we were God's special children because of our deafness. My mother said she wanted to spit at him for saying that.

Because of this, perhaps — and the fact that she didn't like getting up early in the morning — she permitted my 5-year-old brother to walk the eight blocks by himself to catch the school bus each day. By the time he was 6, he would take me by the hand and escort me to the bus station and then to my preschool class. I adored and looked up to my brother, whom I trusted implicitly, not realizing the immense responsibility that was being placed on his shoulders. He was older and so much smarter then me. Even though we set ourselves up as intense rivals, we forged a unique bond.

Sibling rivalry did occur, however. My mother kept in touch with a psychologist named Miriam Fiedler who wrote a book about the pilot program in which were involved.* "When they go to bed at night, each one can find a dozen excuses for calling me," my mother wrote to Ms. Fiedler at one point. "Of course, there is always water and who gets it first. Even if I go with two glasses and give my

> My parents came to understand that good amplification and optimal use of residual hearing was our ticket to the 'hearing' world.

---

* Fiedler, M. F. (1952). *Deaf Children in a Hearing World: Their Education and Adjustment.* New York: The Ronald Press Co.

daughter one glass first, then my son who is older has a little tantrum. Sometimes my children delight in teasing each other. For example, my daughter cups her hands over her mouth and whispers to me, excluding her brother. Then, of course, my son is frustrated because he just does not know how to get a look in, and my daughter won't let me tell him what the secret is . . . and he cries because he wants me to tell him. But he will do the same thing to her."

Quite honestly, I remember very little of my preschool years. I vaguely recall happy times both at school and at home playing with friends from our building and neighborhood. In 1948, we bought our first TV (the black-and-white ones had just come on the market) and I loved watching and listening to Howdy Doody, Clarabell the Clown, and Buffalo Bob from the old "Howdy Doody Show." I remember many happy experiences growing up in our two-room apartment in a Bronx tenement, playing on our fire escape or in the building elevator with my best friend; going down the block to the candy store where neat things could be bought for a penny or nickel; and going across the street to play in the schoolyard with the other children. I also remember many times playing with my mother and listening to her talk about a variety of topics. She read books to me every day, and I always enjoyed those quiet times. I don't recall her ever making a big issue out of my hearing loss.

When my family took weekend trips, I fondly recall the many songs we sang in the car. As we learned more songs, we would sing them in rounds, particularly those that were repetitive such as "Three Blind Mice," "Row, Row, Row Your Boat," and "Brother John" (as well as its French version, "Frère Jacques"). It was great fun keeping up with my parents' rhythm and tempo while putting their words in the background so I could sing different words.

> My brother and I were not mollycoddled by our parents. Despite their best planning, they knew we would be puzzled when some children rebuffed us.

I vividly recall one incident involving my brother that occurred when he was playing outside one weekend. My mother looked out of our second floor window and saw that several big boys were picking on him. She immediately told my father, who calmly put on his shoes and went downstairs. He separated the bullies and told them it was not fair for all of them to gang up on my brother. My father, a former Golden Gloves boxer, suggested that in the future they should fight him one at a time. Then, when the older boys left, my father started teaching my brother how to fight so he could adequately defend himself.

My brother and I were not mollycoddled or overprotected by our parents. Perhaps this is what my mother was thinking when she reportedly said: "Even though we as parents plan wisely and do all we can to attract playmates for our children, they are going to be unhappy and puzzled when some children rebuff them."

Grade School, Ownership, and Play

My mother was apprehensive about sending me off to the neighborhood school just up the block. When all was said and done, however, I did remarkably well in first grade. My teacher, in fact, never stopped raving about me. At that time, I talked incessantly and knew many stories, songs, and poems — and "at the drop of a hat, would recite them all."

All I can remember about the first grade is that I was the shortest girl in my class, so I liked the shortest boy in the class, and I loved recess when we would play outside, particularly when that boy and I were able to play with each other.

By the time I completed first grade, my mother wrote, "I was always under the impression that without me my children would be lost, that I had to be their ears, nursemaid, interpreter, constant companion, etc. I found out I was wrong, and I am glad. Ellen talks and talks and talks, and her teachers think she is doing very well. She's easily understood now, very independent, has a strong will, tries awfully hard to get her way, but she's learning to give in too."

It was at this point that deafness began taking a back seat in our family life. My mother considered her "job" done in that my brother and I were using our hearing aids well, we had no problems communicating with anyone, and we were attending local schools. So, she went back to work full time, making sure that we had cookies and milk, chocolate pudding, or gelatin waiting for us at the end of each school day.

My family moved from the Bronx to Queens the summer before I entered second grade. I was finally able to sleep in a regular bed since having to sleep in a crib until the end of first grade was beginning to embarrass me. From this point, I remember much more of my elementary school years. My transition to another neighborhood school was seamless and I did well, encountering no academic problems in any of my subjects. Although my vocabulary was so-so compared to my peers, it was considered mediocre in my family because my brother rose above the norm. In fact, he was already reading the entire sports sections of the daily newspapers.

> Although my vocabulary was so-so compared to my peers, it was considered mediocre in my family because my brother rose above the norm.

Although homework was not a significant part of my school experience, I did a great deal of reading at home. I loved to read comic books in the bathroom and with a flashlight under my blanket in bed. I would also read the backs of cereal boxes while eating breakfast, and a variety of children's books at all hours of the day. Spelling came effortlessly to me, which is why I placed second in my school spelling bee without studying.

The best part of growing up was playing. Each school year, I had at least one best friend along with other girlfriends from my neighborhood. Every day, we made dates to play — and play we did! We played every game imaginable, from "stoop ball" to "hit the penny" to "monkey in the middle." We jumped rope, rode our bikes, played hide and seek, attended Brownie and Girl Scout meetings, went to art and ballet and toe dancing classes, took accordion lessons, and competed in Nok-Hockey® and table tennis. Our neighborhood was full of children, and I remember always having a good time.

As a family, we took many weekend car trips. We played all kinds of verbal games that facilitated our continually expanding knowledge of geography, spelling, and trivia. I have no doubt that these games helped instill in me a lifelong habit of listening and learning, although I think my parents probably played these games just to keep my brother and me from fighting.

I do remember some unhappy times at home, however — either as a result of fighting with my brother or being disciplined by my father. Just as my mother was the dominant figure during my language-learning years, my father was a powerful figure in my character-forming years. He was a strong individual: mentally, emotionally, and physically. As soon as he returned from the Korean War, he made it his priority to provide financially for his family so our important needs would be met. Regardless of cost, every two years my brother and I were always given the best and latest hearing aids. My father also ensured that we were given 100% of his emotional support when we strived to make anything happen. Although I didn't appreciate it at the time, I encountered his strong will early on.

When it came to managing our behavior, my father often said, "Teaching young children how to behave is no different than teaching dogs how to behave." He tolerated neither disrespect nor poor behavior from either of his children. While I vividly recall the intense rivalry and frequent physical fighting that escalated between my brother and me during our grade school years, the moment we heard that my father was nearing home, we immediately stopped. Although my father never hit me, I knew better than to cross him.

In fourth grade, I was about to go to my best friend's birthday party and my mother said I needed to cut my nails. I refused and was on my way out the door when my father ordered me not to leave the house until I had done so. Grounded like stone, fury overtook me and I silently sulked. Because of my stubborn pride, I chose to forego the birthday party and, of course, I eventually had to cut my nails in order to leave our apartment the next day.

My hearing loss remained largely a nonissue. I simply carried my hearing aid batteries everywhere I went. Ever since first grade, knowing when and how to change my batteries was solely my responsibility. In fact, all I had to do was let my mother know when my supply was running low and she would buy some more. The only time I recall being conscious of my hearing loss was when I saw a second grade class photo. How conspicuous that body-worn aid was on the front of my blouse! From that point, I always wore my aid under my blouses. Fortunately, the following school year, behind-the-ear hearing aids were developed. My brother and I were probably among the first American children to each have our own BTE hearing aids. I remember a sense of freedom with no more cords, no more harness, no more anything on my chest!

Each time we bought a new hearing aid, I had a choice in the decision-making process. Knowing instinctively which aid was better for me, I would argue with any hearing aid dealer or audiologist who disagreed when I said the ear mold didn't fit properly or my hearing aid didn't work the way it should. My parents trusted in how I heard and would not accept others denying my feelings.

For a short while in fourth grade, a speech teacher came to visit me on a weekly basis. She wanted to teach me how to produce a *ch* sound. In isolation, I couldn't really hear the difference between *sh* and *ch* except that the latter

> The only time I recall being conscious of my hearing loss was when I saw a second grade class photo. How conspicuous that body-worn aid was.

seemed to be said more quickly. After a few weeks, she decided to show me the difference in print, and when I saw *tsh*, I suddenly realized why the *ch* sounded different and immediately began saying *ch* correctly. That was the last time I saw the speech teacher. I didn't like being pulled out of the classroom for any reason whatsoever. If I needed speech therapy from that point on, it would have to be on Saturdays.

Although my language skills were as good as those of my friends, I mispronounced a few words every so often, and these soon became family jokes. For example, when I read *Treasure Island* for the first time, I had never heard anyone say that second word before. So, when I said "island" for the first time, I said "iz-land" rather than "eye-lind" and that would bring laughter from my brother and parents. These mispronunciations would become part of our family lore. I had no choice but to learn how to laugh at myself.

Middle Grades, Experiments, and Happiness

What a glorious time I had during my junior high years! Almost from the outset of seventh grade, I developed two new best friends. For the next three years, we were known as "The Three Musketeers." We were so close and yet we each also had a secondary circle of friends. I had three other good friends and traveled in a different social circle with each of them. With one friend, I played the role of a beatnik and associated with those who smoked marijuana, played jazz, and rode motorcycles. With other friends, I joined the world of teenage hoods with ducktails and black leather clothes, smoking cigarettes and congregating on street corners. With still others, I traversed the world of typical naive but exuberantly wild suburban do-gooders who went ice skating and played volleyball, hanging out in ice-cream parlors. All in all, they provided wonderful learning experiences, and I fondly recall all those friendships — complete with the dumb experiences and secrets we shared.

Whether I actually was or not, I felt like a typical preteen. My weekends were full and I was interested in meeting boys. And meet boys we did — all over Queens and Manhattan. I was limited only by the night curfews imposed by my parents. Had they known where I was going, however, they likely would have limited my travels.

I talked on the phone incessantly to all my friends, so much so that my parents got me my own telephone line. Nevertheless, there were repeated father-daughter contests of wills. One evening, for example, my father told me to get off the phone because I had been on it for hours. "OK, daddy, I will — just gimme a minute," I said. More than just one minute passed and I was again told to get off the phone. When my father came back a third time, he literally pulled the phone cord out of the socket and I was without a phone for weeks until I apologized and agreed not to abuse my privileges again.

Being a good student was not on my list of priorities. I was interested only in my friends and having fun. Somehow, I learned enough of whatever was taught to obtain B and C grades, although I was given countless homework assignments in which I had to write anywhere from 1,000 to 5,000 times: *I will not talk in class.* I certainly learned how to write with teeny tiny handwriting and to use every available space of paper while riding the bus to and from school each day.

The only time in my school career that I asked my mother to assist me with homework was to review my written reports and essays. She continually complained about my wordiness, my run-on sentences, and my tendency to obfuscate. She clearly disliked getting involved in my schoolwork, but she always tried to help me improve my written English by encouraging me to write shorter sentences with less flourish.

I don't recall whether my hearing loss presented any significant issues for me while I was a preteen, although I did avoid swimming because I didn't want to remove my hearing aid. Not hearing was not an option for me. I remember a few very unpleasant moments outside in the winter when my hearing aid battery froze and I couldn't hear.

The fact that I used a hearing aid didn't seem to affect my friendships with anyone, either boy or girl. That belief was confirmed by my father when I lamented that I probably didn't have a date for the junior high prom because of my hearing loss. His retort made a lot of sense to me: "That is probably not true. It is likely due to your lack of long-term friendships with boys and they don't know you. Maybe the ones that do know you just don't like you." He then discussed how we tend to magnify things when we are kids, and used his short height as an example. He helped me realize that everyone has some imperfection that creates a sense of inadequacy — even something like a pimple on the nose can do this to an adolescent.

> My father helped me realize that everyone has some imperfection that creates a sense of inadequacy – even something like a pimple can do this.

I stopped speech therapy after grade school since there was no longer a need for it. I was perfectly intelligible to everyone, though most strangers I met thought I had an accent. I do recall one incident when I was talking about a "dick-chin-AIRee" to some friends on the school bus and detected some smirking and subtle snickering. After school that day, I found out from my mother how to correctly pronounce "dictionary," and since then I have made a special point to learn the correct pronunciation of all new words. Of course, my mother was quite good about correcting my mispronunciations in private.

There was no such thing as an assistive listening system while I was in school. I used my hearing aid and, of my own volition, would generally choose to sit toward the front of the room — often the second row from where the teacher typically stood so I could hear as well as get a good visual scan of most of my classmates.

Although I still fought frequently and sometimes bitterly with my brother, he now traveled in different circles than I did. Because he had skipped a grade, he was attending the local high school while I was in junior high. Yet I remember and cherish those few private conversations we had when we commiserated about our hearing loss. It was important to know that I was not alone in my intense dislike for those who would exaggerate their lip movements when they learned about our hearing loss. Both of us intensely disliked pity, and we had no patience for sympathy. It seemed as though we had identical experiences when it came to our hearing difficulties and hearing aids — that was the tie that bound us and would never be broken, regardless of our arguments.

High School, Failures, and Anonymity

I joined a high school sorority composed of diversely interesting girls who did not meet the established norm. Being popular in my circle of friends was very important to me, certainly more so than doing well academically. My high school years included all my good friends from junior high plus my sorority sisters — so many friends and not enough time to spend with all of them! Therefore, I did what had to be done: I cut a few days of school here and there, neglected to do much of my homework, and didn't particularly pay much attention in my classes.

In my first year of high school, a math teacher once called on me to answer a question. As usual, I was busy talking with one of my friends. When I heard him call my name, I turned around to face him and said, "What? I'm sorry, I did not hear your question." The teacher became angry and yelled, "What's the matter with you, are you deaf or something?" I was absolutely mortified that he would say such a thing in front of my classmates.

Later that day when my mother came home from work, I recounted the incident to her in teary-eyed fashion. She shed a few tears, too, and said she would talk to the teacher the next day to demand an apology from him. A bit later, however, we recounted the story for my father while we were eating dinner and his reaction was quite different. He told my mother not to butt in and said that I should apologize to the teacher instead. My father was angry at me! He said that because I was talking in class, the teacher had every right to be upset with me. He also reminded me that there were 5,000 students in my high school and it was highly unlikely the teacher even knew about my hearing loss.

> Angry that I was not paying attention, a teacher yelled, 'What's the matter with you, are you deaf or something?' I was mortified.

Since I had neither homework nor studying on my agenda, my grades suffered. Unfortunately, by the time I completed the 10th grade, I had also failed a couple of courses. Getting F's was a rather unpleasant reality that meant there would be consequences. My parents were typical second-generation Americans who fit the middle-class mold, so it had long been drilled into my psyche that I was going to college. I had been raised to be responsible for myself and to bear the consequences of my actions. Even though I knew my parents would always provide me with emotional and moral support, it was of little solace when I had to attend summer school. That was a rude awakening! It was clear that most of the other kids who went to summer school were on a general or vocational track and certainly not destined for college. Pride reared its head and I buckled down to study. Failure indeed proved instructive.

However, upon returning to high school as a sophomore, I again got caught up with all my friends. My trials with different lifestyles continued: the college preppies, the pseudo-intelligentsia, the disenfranchised — all were fodder for my inquisitive and flexible nature. I continued day and night forays to the Greenwich Village jazz clubs, Washington Square, Lincoln Center film festivals, assorted parks in Queens, Columbia and New York University pubs, as well as basement sorority and fraternity weekend parties. I had a smashing time!

Meanwhile, my relationship with my parents suffered. I was somewhat out of control and rebelled against any rules imposed on me. My father and I butted heads more than once. On one occasion, when I said something disrespectful to my father, my mother suggested that I apologize to him. I refused and wouldn't talk to him, which meant, of course, that I couldn't ask him for my allowance. Pride again got in my way, and I went without an allowance for 9 months! Finally, I broke down and apologized — a high school kid without money is essentially grounded. This had been another classic contest of wills that I ultimately lost. My father's indomitable will always proved stronger than mine.

Yet, there were times when I got along well with my father. He gave me my first summer job at the age of 16, in between my sophomore and junior years. I worked as an entry-level secretary for an executive in his mutual fund business. I had to answer the phone and take messages, take dictation and then type up letters, as well as filing and collating papers. For the first time, I found something not easy. My hearing loss got in the way. Some callers spoke with accents and others mumbled. Sweating through some of those telephone conversations, I messed up quite a few messages. When I was called into the executive's office so he could dictate a letter, I quickly learned the value of shorthand (which I didn't know), and I sweated even more through several words that I didn't understand. Fast dictation does not go well with lipreading! That summer, I also learned the meaning of words such as "ramification" and "diversification." My new best friend was a dictionary.

> In my first summer job as a secretary for an executive, I found something not easy for the first time. My hearing loss got in the way.

From that experience, I learned that my father was right — that I needed to go to college. As the school year wound down that spring, I had told him I was thinking of quitting high school, so he laid out the pros and cons. When he showed me the expense side, such as me having to pay him rent, I quickly grasped the importance of a good salary. Unlike my very intelligent but more emotionally inclined mother, my father was an extraordinarily logical, street-smart, calm, and persistent individual who always could successfully appeal to my reason.

For my final two years of high school, I had a part-time job as cashier in a supermarket. Instead of getting an allowance from my father, I had to pay him a portion of my wages to share in the expenses of living in their home. Of course, I didn't know until later that my father was simply saving my money for me. Early on, I learned the value of a buck.

Throughout high school, I was always physically active. Table tennis and crafts were easy for me; biking from Queens to Greenwich Village always gave me a wonderful sense of accomplishment; going to museums and playing with a Frisbee were terrific ways to meet older boys; ice skating and skiing were enjoyable challenges. The only sport I avoided was swimming since I wanted to hear other people at all times. Although I frequently went to the movies, I knew I missed a good bit of the dialogue, and that is why I gravitated toward foreign films. With subtitles, I even understood the subtle nuances spoken by each character.

At some point during my senior year, I met with a vocational rehabilitation counselor because I wanted financial assistance for college. After taking a series of aptitude tests, it was agreed that I was college material, but I was dissuaded from a variety of professions, including teaching. He argued that I should become a librarian because hearing well was not necessary for that job. I was upset, to say the least, and when I told my father, he was furious! He convinced me that I could be and do anything that I wanted if I was willing to work hard enough for it.

In the last semester of my senior year, I heard from someone I had not seen since my preschool years. I remembered that this friend had also had success wearing hearing aids despite a significant hearing loss. She invited me to a party at her home and, curious to meet her after 15 years, I accepted the invitation. I had my father drive me there — about a half an hour after her party began. When I walked downstairs into her basement, I was stunned. All the boys and girls were dancing and signing to each other! Then the music stopped, but everyone kept dancing. I was directed to the girl who was my preschool friend and tried to make conversation with her, but I didn't know sign language. It was hopelessly frustrating. Barely an hour had passed when I tearfully phoned my father, asking him to pick me up as soon as possible.

I was just devastated by my old friend's world, which was so foreign to me. As soon as I told my father about this party, however, I put it out of my mind and didn't think about it for another five years.

I graduated from high school with a C average. Interestingly, by this time, tests showed that I had attained a vocabulary and reading level significantly above my peers with normal hearing, although this certainly wasn't because of my attention to schoolwork! Clearly, my love of reading was the reason.

The summer following graduation, my father and I began forging a closer and different kind of relationship. He was teaching me how to drive and had given me a second summer job as a secretary — but this time I worked for him since he had become president of a financial planning company. Because I was the assistant to his secretary, she bailed me out when I messed up phone messages. The rest of my job was easy. I drove my dad to work and home every day; he entrusted his life and car to me as I drove him from eastern Queens to Wall Street in Manhattan. He was rapidly becoming the most important mentor in my life.

Colleges, Responsibilities, and Freedom

Because of my mediocre academic record, I didn't apply to competitive colleges. Instead, for my freshman year, I attended Pace University in New York City. I chose Pace because it was business-oriented and there were seven boys for every girl enrolled. While I took an intense dislike to accounting, a freshman English professor helped me see my creative writing possibilities, which provided the impetus for my love affair with a thesaurus. Thus, I began writing my collection of more than a hundred poems.

The summer after my freshman year of college, I served as a counselor in a sleep-away camp for children with orthopedic disabilities. One cute little camper, Anthony, had muscular dystrophy (like many of the other children). But he was also hard of hearing. I was drawn to him like a magnet. I think this was my first inkling of what was to come.

I then applied to Keuka College, a small Christian women's school in upstate New York, thinking I might like living in a dormitory (away from home!) and having access to the all-men's colleges nearby. At this college, all students were required to complete a two-month winter internship. I chose to do mine at an oral day school for the deaf in Manhattan. This purposeful foray into the world of children who were deaf was rather intriguing.

Nevertheless, I was one of only seven Jewish women at Keuka, and the experience of attending a sequestered Christian college proved to be an unwanted eye-opener for someone raised in such a diverse city as New York. There had been about 5,000 children in my high school — 1,000-plus in my graduating class alone — yet the entire student body at Keuka comprised fewer than 500 girls, so I planned to transfer elsewhere for my junior year. I had also gotten caught up in the social world of all-night card games and weekend fraternity parties, and my grades continued to be mediocre.

From there, having been accepted to UCLA's summer school, I went to Los Angeles. I wanted to go west, but it proved to be somewhat of an unsavory experience. The more significant limitation of my deafness reared its ugly head for the first time. I was taking two philosophy courses in a huge auditorium five mornings a week, and seating was on a first-come, first-served basis. There were more than 250 students for each class, unlike anything I had experienced before. There was no way I could understand anything the professors said. So I stopped trying after a few days and started cutting classes.

Instead, I spent my afternoons in Tarzana learning to be a trapeze artist, with the half-baked notion that I might one day join the circus or hitchhike to Alaska. My weekends were spent in San Francisco with the flower children of the '60s. Before the summer was over, I knew my parents would be returning from their European vacation and I had to face the music. I hitched a ride home and, upon their return to New York, they heard me out. I expected them to react quite negatively, but to my surprise my father seemed to be somewhat understanding. I think he instinctively realized what had occurred to me and simply chalked it up as an expensive learning experience.

There was no way I could understand anything the professors said, so I stopped trying after a few days and started cutting classes.

For my junior and senior years, I attended Oglethorpe University in Atlanta, and was actually a pretty good student. I finally had some direction in my life — someplace in the education field. Classes were relatively small, so I majored in elementary education. I also dated extensively, and again my hearing loss didn't seem to be an issue. After a year, I met someone from the Midwest and became seriously involved almost immediately. Initially, beause of his midwestern twang I had some difficulties understanding him on the phone, but that soon passed. Eventually, we made plans to get married.

In college, I joined the fencing and rifle shooting clubs, but curtailed fencing after a few months because the mask prevented me from understanding instructions and conversations around me. I lived in an off-campus apartment, so my roommates all knew that I needed to wake up with a vibrating alarm clock. They often borrowed it on important test days.

The summer between my junior and senior years, I worked in New York as a proofreader. This necessitated my listening well to a coworker who would read press releases. Needless to say, I preferred that she do the listening while I did the reading, but we always took turns. I simply made sure that she sat on my hearing aid side when she was reading the press releases. That summer experience gave me much confidence in knowing written language composition.

For my college graduation present, my parents gave me a summer in Europe. The year was 1967 and college students were hitchhiking all over the continent. Who was I to be any different? For the first half of the summer, I traveled with one of the friends I had grown up with in New York. She was fluent in French, so we met in Paris and she showed me the ropes. By the time we left France and she returned to the States, I was comfortable with a solitary life on the European road. Again, I was having a grand old time with all the good-looking young men I was meeting — musicians, students, sailors, waiters. No one even asked me about my accent. Hearing loss an issue? As long as I had a battery in my knapsack, I was fine.

Graduate School, True Knowledge, and Perseverance

Reality intruded when it was time for me to return to the United States. It was important to me that my parents like the man I planned to marry — and they did. They recognized his kindness, compassion, and sincere and friendly nature. Most of all, they were so pleased that he adored me. Indeed, the man I married was a wonderful supporter of whatever I wanted to do with my life, and that helped me greatly during graduate school.

Because of the Vietnam War, my husband's Air Force reserve unit was reactivated, so we spent a year in Charleston, South Carolina. While he worked at the base in Charleston, I found a part-time job similar to the one I had in college: a saleswoman in a department store. My husband spent the following year in Vietnam, so I put my degree to good use by teaching at a private kindergarten in New York. In the evenings, I took graduate classes on the education of children with neurological impairments.

We moved back to Atlanta as soon as my husband returned stateside. I spoke to the head of the graduate department of communication disorders at Emory University about becoming a student there. He dissuaded me and suggested that since I spoke so well I might instead consider being a subject in their experiments. Insulted and angered, I wouldn't have bothered to return except for my husband, who urged me to formally apply as a student the following year. I taught elementary school for one more year, and then found out that my formal application to Emory had been accepted. I'm sure it helped that the department had a new director who was unaware of my hearing loss.

Happily, but with trepidation, I started taking courses in audiology, speech, and deaf education for the next two years. From the outset, a senior professor made it very clear that she felt I was out of my element and should not be in their graduate program. Needless to say, one of my first courses was "Phonetics," given by this same professor. This meant that after I learned the International Phonetic Alphabet, I would listen to the professor say unfamiliar words and phonetically transcribe those nonsense words (like a spelling test of new vocabulary, but without the benefit of sentences). Talk about difficult listening experiences! That first quarter, I did a lot of listening, watching, writing, and sweating — all at the same time. I passed the course without receiving any latitude from that professor. In retrospect that Phonetics course would have been so much easier had I been able to use an assistive listening system.

Getting a C in Phonetics was the lowest grade I received in graduate school. The rest of my grades were mostly A's, with a few B's. Having taken that course, my confidence level was high and I sailed through graduate training. The same professor also taught a Psycholinguistics class the following quarter, and she noted that she had never had another graduate student understand or write on the subject as well as I did.

Upon taking my first audiology course, I quickly learned that my brother and I were officially "deaf." I remember calling my brother to share this insight. This was quite a revelation because all these years I had assumed we were both hard of hearing — at least, that was the term my parents used. In my audiology course, I learned the power of expectations and what great damage can be done to individuals by labeling. The label of "deafness" stung.

> I learned the power of expectations and what great damage can be done to individuals by labeling. The label of 'deafness' stung.

"Psychology of Deafness" was another of my first-year graduate courses. I read a classic textbook by a renowned author in the field and was astounded that so many people believed in stereotypical nonsense. In fact, I joked with my brother about certain "facts" I had read in that classic textbook: that he shook his leg because he was deaf; that his reading level could not possibly be so much better than that of his peers; that he could not possibly process things cognitively at an abstract level. I found much of what I read in that book to be demeaning and insulting. So much for the "psychology of deafness"!

Another of my first-year courses dealt with teaching language to children who were deaf. Again, I was dumbfounded. No wonder children who were deaf were illiterate and couldn't master spoken language! I was a linguistically competent graduate student and yet I didn't know an adjective from an adverb; nor did I remember what prepositions were — I must have cut those classes when that grammar was taught in grade school. I couldn't believe my professors were convinced that this information was important for children who were deaf to develop natural spoken language.

Still another first-year course was "Teaching Speech to Deaf Children." Since grade school, I knew that my *r* sounded like a *w*, which I attributed to the fact I couldn't hear the difference between them. Therefore, I made a habit of avoiding words that began with the *r* sound. Now, it was time to face my speech demons. If I was going to help children improve their speech, I figured I should first know how to properly say all the English sounds myself. So, after consulting the textbooks, I decided the best way to learn how to say *r* was to curl my tongue upward and backward just as the pictures showed. Lo and behold, I realized that I couldn't do this with my tongue. My frenulum (the piece of skin that connects the tongue to the floor of the mouth) hurt when I tried to do that. I had never bothered to elevate my tongue any higher than needed for producing the *t*, *d*, or *l* sounds. I practiced doing this for weeks. My husband thought I was nuts, but my tongue gradually became stretched out and more elevated — without causing me pain. Then I learned the party trick of how to squirt saliva from those two tiny holes at the base of my frenulum. From that point on, it was just persistent motivation to articulate precisely every time I said a word that began with *r*.

All in all, completing my first year of graduate courses represented a milestone in my life . . . and there was no turning back. I made a decision to take on the challenge of proving these professors wrong in more ways than one. Because my grades were excellent, except for that Phonetics course, I was given a full fellowship for my second year.

My second year at Emory was relatively easy — mostly a bunch of audiological and teaching practica at various hospital and school sites. I gained experience working with children and adults of all ages. Just as important, I finally read Fiedler's book *Deaf Children in a Hearing World*, which focused on 12 children with hearing loss (including my brother and me) who had participated in that New York preschool pilot project in the 1940s. I was just learning what made us different from others who were deaf: we heard, we listened, we spoke, and we fitted into the mainstream with ease — or so I thought. This opened up more private conversations with my brother. It was then that I learned that how he felt about his deafness was not quite the same as how I felt about mine.

> I came to realize the paths chosen for us by our parents have far-reaching effects, and some of these opportunities are beyond our making.

First, my brother's deafness was greater than mine (he had a 95 dB loss in one ear, and the other was essentially nonresponsive to sound). Second, he didn't start using a hearing aid until he was 4½ years old, and until then he was taught how to speak primarily by lipreading. He attended special oral classes for children who were deaf until completing the third grade, and he had skipped the second grade because he was clearly the "star" of all his classes. When he was mainstreamed in the fourth grade, it was during the "sink or swim" atmosphere of the 1950s, meaning that no support services were available. I learned that he secretly adopted the persona of Superman/Clark Kent — the latter identity was for attending school. Clearly the more intelligent of the two of us, he had more painful issues to deal with, and I felt deeply for him.

What I learned about my brother unquestionably influenced how I would come to approach parents and people with hearing loss. I came to fully realize that the paths chosen for us by our parents have far-reaching effects on our lives, and that some of these opportunities are beyond our making.

Given that I was an anomaly in 1970 — perhaps the only "hearing deaf" teacher for "oral deaf" kids that year — doors opened for me. Never again would I need to apply for a job. Several months before I received my master's degree in deaf education/audiology, I was invited by the director of special education at a local school system to work as a teacher for primary grade school children with hearing loss within a special oral classroom setting.

Career Choice, a Renewed Mission, and Anticipation

For the next four years, I worked as a preschool and primary grade teacher in public and private oral self-contained classrooms. All the while, I attended graduate school in the evenings and obtained a Specialist in Education degree. My extensive coursework in special education administration and supervision enabled me to earn an Ed.S. designation from Georgia State University. Although I was a relatively inexperienced teacher, it surprised me how little my colleagues understood about how to manage hearing aids. Even more puzzling, however, was why many children in my classes were not performing like me.

As a teacher of the deaf, I was acutely aware of the need to hear as effectively as possible so I used a body-worn hearing aid while on the job. That trusty old powerful device from grade school still worked well for me! During that time, the schools used me for publicity — *the deaf teaching the deaf how to talk*. It made good newspaper copy.

In my third year of teaching children who were deaf, I became acquainted with Doreen Pollack and learned that the lifestyle my parents had chosen for my brother and me was one she had advocated since the 1940s. Pollack was the clinician we had met at Columbia Presbyterian Hospital some 20 years earlier — the lady my mother thought was a "quack" — who had become famous for her pioneering efforts as an Auditory-Verbal therapist. After talking with her, I realized that what my own parents had done was remarkable in that they essentially opted for an auditory-based educational road paved with natural language and speech, based on plain common sense. However, they didn't have the benefit of an Auditory-Verbal professional to guide them. I soon devoured Doreen's most recent book and it changed me forever. When I discussed the activities presented in the book with my mother, she remembered trying variations of them with me just because they seemed like common sense. From that point, I was done with self-contained classrooms. I wanted to enable other parents to travel the same path that mine had. With every fiber of my being, I knew that parents were the key to bridging the abyss of deafness, not professionals. There was no better way to pay tribute to my parents than to make this my professional mission.

> I realized that what my own parents had done was remarkable in that they essentially opted for for an auditory-based educational road.

As always, my husband supported my career and was proud of what I was doing, even though I worked long hours. We had spoken frequently of having a child, but I kept delaying it because I didn't want to bring any more children with hearing loss into the world. Although there was no proof that my deafness was genetic, intuition and common sense told me it was. Ultimately, however, I was ready to have a child because I knew that I had learned how to effectively deal with any child's hearing loss.

For the next two years, I established an Auditory-Verbal program at a private oral school for children in Atlanta, serving as the program's parent–infant coordinator. It was a rewarding period of my life, and I confidently implemented all the A-V strategies I had read about in Doreen's book as well as those my mother had worked on with me! The infants and toddlers in the program learned to hear and speak rather effortlessly, just like me. I was so pleased, but I was also frustrated because some of these children were going to enter the school's self-contained preschool classrooms where a "washout effect" might occur over time. I felt that the learned listening and natural speech skills acquired would begin to sound "deafy" when these children were educated full time with other children who were deaf. I knew it was time for me to think of another way to attain my long-term professional goal.

Meanwhile, I moved up to the doctoral program at Georgia State specializing in infancy and family therapy, again helped financially by fellowships, I also was expecting a baby! Unfortunately, on the same day I learned I was pregnant, my husband decided to start a business that would keep him away from home six days a week. This was the beginning of the end of our marriage since ongoing honest communication had been the bedrock of our relationship.

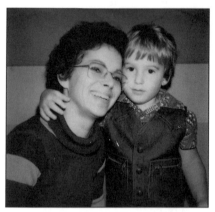

I was concerned by my son's sketchy hearing at an early age, caused by the ear infection otitis media. *After extensive surgery to correct the effects of the infection, he could hear normally.*

A Child, Forced Knowledge, and Anger

My beautiful and healthy son was born in 1975. And, just like my mother with my brother 30 years earlier, I doted on him. There was one big difference, however: I immediately had his hearing tested in the hospital, and then frequently thereafter. I knew he listened to me when I used natural, melodic language. By the time he was 1, his comprehension of spoken language was outstanding, but I was still puzzled by his hearing. Sometimes he seemed not to hear as well as on other days. Since he was 5 months old, he had been continuously on some kind of antibiotic for the middle ear infection known as *otitis media*.

I carefully scanned the literature on *otitis media*, learning that this was a hot topic among otologists in the mid-1970s. Dr. Charles Bluestone, considered a maverick in this area at the time, was advocating assertive medical management for children with repeated middle ear pathology. The literature was beginning to show a correlation between those with auditory memory difficulties and those with a history of *otitis media*. Armed with this knowledge, I angrily confronted my son's pediatrician of two years and asked him why he was repeatedly treating my son in a passive manner — particularly knowing that he was at genetic risk for hearing loss. Needless to say, he became quite defensive, arguing that ear infections were the most common and routine disease of any pediatrician's daily caseload.

I then took my 2-year-old to an otologist to have his hearing checked again. This time, test results showed a bilateral 75 dB conductive hearing loss! After my tears of recrimination subsided, I took immediate action. A date for surgery was scheduled so that a tonsillectomy, adenoidectomy, and tympanostomy could all be done at the same time. Immediately after the surgery, during which much thick, green, smelly gook was removed from my son's middle ears, he could once again hear normally. However, though his receptive language was excellent, his speech was more like that of an 18-month-old child — with many substitutions and omissions. I decided to personally provide intensive Auditory-Verbal therapy every day after I returned home from work. It worked like a charm, and within 6 months his speech and expressive language had demonstrated more than 12 months of growth. To say that I was thrilled when strangers marveled at how beautifully he spoke was an understatement. As Jewish moms are wont to say, I "kvelled"!

From that point, assertive management of middle ear infections was a focal point of my mission in educating parents. I sent my son's pediatrician a long letter presenting a great deal of data on the relationship between auditory memory, speech and language development, and history of *otitis media*. We argued a bit about the need to pay better attention to these children, and because he didn't agree with me, I switched pediatricians.

For my doctoral dissertation, I decided to focus on finding a relationship between recurrent *otitis media* during infancy and subsequent auditory memory performance.

An A-V Center, Accomplishments, and Sacrifices

In 1977, a teaching colleague and I decided to establish a nonprofit A-V center in Atlanta. We called it the Auditory Education Center and conducted therapy with our first "client" in the lobby of an office building on Saturdays. Then we rented space in a church. As the first year progressed, however, it became clear that my colleague was increasingly busy with her own growing family, so the continued existence, growth, and leadership of the center (known today as the Auditory-Verbal Center of Atlanta) was left with me. For the first three years, I didn't pay myself a salary because I knew the center would need to build capital in order to receive grant monies. I wrote a proposal for a federal grant as a doctoral course project and the U.S. Department of Education agreed to fund the center, meaning I could have the model program that I wanted.

At this time, I was also scheduled to embark on a year-long research project while in the middle of divorce proceedings and having to deal with a 3-year-old about to begin preschool. Although I had completed all the doctoral coursework, the written exam, and the prospectus for my dissertation, I knew there wouldn't be time to spend on the dissertation if I was to effectively direct the pilot project at the A-V center and still be a good mother. I decided to give up on my doctorate and haven't looked back once.

The $300,000 three-year grant from the DOE was really the start of many follow-up activities. First, it enabled me to hire administrative and clinical staff. This, in turn, necessitated training and supervision. It was a full-service program, and parents had to participate in an intensive parent counseling/education series of meetings that I facilitated. I established a semiannual assessment protocol that mandated no child receive therapy services without baseline language data. I also established a local board of directors and a professional advisory board that included highly esteemed master A-V clinicians. Finally, I developed a long-term public relations/community education/marketing and fundraising plan of action.

The number of families we served increased slowly each year. The fundraising plan of action was fulfilled and the center became a line item in the state budget and a special ongoing project of its statewide service clubs. In addition, after two rejections, the United Way finally accepted my proposal for the center to become a member agency. So, within a year of completion of the federal grant, the center had a secure and diverse financial base.

Three members of the center's advisory board were my clinical mentors: Dr. Ciwa Griffiths, Helen H. Beebe, and Doreen Pollack. When Helen Beebe came to visit in 1977, she provided honest feedback on several levels. She also suggested that I personally try bilateral amplification. I followed her advice, but soon learned that trying to use my residual hearing in a heretofore unused ear was like starting from scratch. All speech sounded like noise to me so, for myself, I abandoned the concept of binaural hearing.

In 1978, Dr. Griffiths invited me to be a speaker at the Second International Conference on Auditory Techniques — my first national presentation. I was nervous because the audience consisted of more than 500 professionals. I rehearsed and, in my father's presence, learned his time-tested Dale Carnegie techniques for addressing large audiences. I must have performed at least adequately since Dr. Griffiths, Doreen, and Helen invited me to join them as central committee directors on the fledgling International Committee for Auditory Verbal Communication (ICAVC). I was honored to be able to work with the three grand dames (and pioneers) of the Auditory-Verbal Approach.

ICAVC was a special committee within the Alexander Graham Bell Association for the Deaf whose central purpose was advocating for Auditory-Verbal remediation of hearing loss, since the professional world of *deaf educators,* speech-language pathologists, and audiologists had, by and large, not yet learned about this approach. The committee members of ICAVC went on to establish an independent organization known as Auditory-Verbal International, Inc. I learned much that was positive from serving on the committee and founding board, but I also learned how much some Auditory-Verbal therapists like to talk and how some consider AVT to be the crème de la crème of all options.

Some professionals who are used to 'teaching the deaf' associate deafness with 'neediness' and adopt the 'savior complex.'

As executive director of the Auditory-Verbal Center of Atlanta for its first 17 years, I hired a variety of people to serve in administrative and clinical positions. It was interesting that only one of those individuals seemed to see me in a different light because of my deafness, and that individual had previously been a teacher of the deaf. It was clear that she didn't particularly enjoy the thought of someone like me serving as her clinical supervisor. Some professionals who are used to "teaching the deaf" associate deafness with "neediness" and adopt the "savior complex."

In the center's early days, obtaining good statewide press coverage was essential to getting the word out about A-V therapy. I had to be willing to hold myself up as a product of this approach — that of a child who was deaf who grew up to become a hearing and speaking adult. Initially, I was very uncomfortable with this role since it placed my hearing loss in the limelight, and particularly since I had never thought of myself as being deaf. Over time and with repeated TV interviews, I have learned how to deal with the often-pejorative label of being "deaf." I also have learned how to be selective when I use such limiting terms.

Certainly, parents with whom I speak say they have always considered their child as a person with a hearing loss and not a "hearing-impaired person." Deafness need not define anyone, no matter how profound the person's deafness — although I did tell parents that I would occasionally and rather conveniently use the label to my advantage, such as when I got a speeding ticket. That is to say, I would burst into tears while explaining to the officer about my deafness and would then assume the mantle of powerlessness and inability to understand what he or she was saying. Sometimes, the police officer would feel sympathy for me and wouldn't issue a ticket. Tales of incidents such as these would often bring humor to our discussions on the semantics of deafness.

Before leaving Atlanta, I received the Metropolitan Atlanta Community Foundation's Program Management Award on behalf of the center, in addition to being personally recognized by the League for the Hard of Hearing in the form of the Nitchie Award in Human Communication. Recognition by the League represented a "full circle" journey for me and my parents (who also attended the award ceremony in New York) since I had gone to the League for speech lessons on Saturdays while in fifth grade.

I also received awards from various civic service clubs both statewide and nationally, but those recognized me for my deafness rather than my professional accomplishments.

Individuals born with a congenital disability, or one acquired soon after birth, can either rise above the disability or let it define them. To my way of thinking, it is wrong to recognize those people with disabilities for what they have accomplished despite their disability. This was clear to me many times when I would read stories about an individual being recognized as the first person who was deaf to accomplish something and I knew that either my brother or I had already done it. My brother, for instance, had been trained and employed by IBM about 15 years before a newspaper article lauded someone else they had just hired as IBM's first employee who was deaf. To me, it makes more sense to have a newspaper article focus on an employee who has achieved something unique who, by the way, happens to be deaf.

I think credit for rising above a disability should go to the parents of the child with the disability. After all, it is the parents who shape the child's journey toward adulthood. My parents chose as normal a life as possible for my brother and me (and for themselves). My mother was involved in an organization for Jewish women, and my father established a senior citizen community program. They exemplified what it is to give back to the community. My brother and I have done likewise.

By the same token, I find it abhorrent for parents of A-V children to credit a professional for their "successes" when the professional does not (and cannot) make it happen without the parents. Parents are the true heroes. Each A-V

> Over time and with repeated TV interviews, I have learned how to deal with the often-pejorative label of being 'deaf.'

professional merely serves as the guide, with the parents either making it happen or not. Primary credit needs to be assigned where it belongs or there is the risk of facilitating the growth of the savior complex by those professionals who perpetuate learned helplessness within the family. My parents' strong belief in determined perseverance, personal will, and common sense enabled my brother and me to accomplish what we did, despite our deafness. Undoubtedly, this is why I consistently laud my parents — they were my best friends, advisors, mentors, and parents. I could not have asked for better.

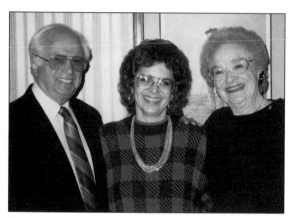

I think credit for rising above a disability should go to the parents of the child with the disability. After all, it is the parents who shape the child's journey toward adulthood. My parents chose as normal a life as possible for my brother and me (and for themselves).

While continuing to develop the A-V center in Atlanta, I transitioned from a painful divorce to once again becoming available on the singles scene. At the same time, I was raising my son and carving a private niche for myself as a local tennis player. I soon met my second significant other and left the social world of dating. My life as executive director seemed to be going well. The development of auditory memory had become an integral part of therapy activities at the center, and the therapists on staff had fully embraced the A-V Approach for the families under our care.

Then my father, the man I revered, was stricken with an illness that brought me to my knees. I flew back and forth from Atlanta to New York every other week during the summer of 1993, focused only on taking care of him. At the same time, there was discord between myself and the board of the A-V center and, after 17 fulfilling years, I chose to resign as executive director.

Relocation, Crises, and Convenient Compassion

Professionals in the field of audiology and education knew I was interested in relocating to another city in either the southeast or southwest United States. I was offered the executive director position at several programs for children with hearing loss. After some consideration, I selected a very small, private oral center in Tampa, Florida. Its board wanted the facility converted to an A-V center, and for the next 6 years I did just that. Before I arrived, its total budget was less than my salary and it served only 10 children; there also was no computer or audiologic equipment. By the time I left in 1998, the center was serving 63 children for both audiology and Auditory-Verbal therapy. A marketing and fundraising plan of action was completed and the center's budget grew to approximately $250,000. In 1996, the center was recognized as Program of the Year by the Alexander Graham Bell Association for the Deaf and Hard of

Hearing, and a therapist I had mentored was named A.G. Bell's Rookie Professional of the Year. Furthermore, Doreen Pollack nominated me for the Beebe Outstanding A-V Clinician of the Year award, given annually by Auditory-Verbal International, which I subsequently won.

However, the stress of my father's slow demise and my transition from one center to another had taken its toll. In January of 1996, while talking on the phone to my father one evening, my world suddenly went silent. I couldn't hear. I told my father, "Daddy, I think my battery died. Hold on a minute." I went to change my battery, perturbed that it had gone out so suddenly since this had never happened before. But when the new battery still didn't seem to work, I was deeply upset. I got back on the phone and told my father, "Daddy, I think my hearing aid died on me. I need to go to the center and get a loaner. I'll call you back later." As I drove to the center, I became increasingly panic-stricken. Something was wrong! No hearing aid at the center worked for me. Somehow, I had instantaneously lost my hearing and the world as I knew it had collapsed.

All I heard, day and night, was the roaring of a subway train. With free-flowing, nonstop tears, I at least had the presence of mind to realize that a cochlear implant was my next step. Having worked with children with implants since 1984, I knew the potential of electrical hearing. I faxed some critical information about this to my parents and they immediately flew to my side, silently grieving with me for what I had lost. I made arrangements for an esteemed cochlear implant surgeon to first try intravenous steroid treatments for a few days in the hospital. That was not successful, and I decided to discontinue the treatment because hospitalization was expensive. I had just changed insurance companies and the new policy excluded coverage on my ear and any hearing disorders for a 6-month period, including my impending cochlear implant surgery. Within a few weeks, I went ahead with the implant in my left ear — the one I had always used for my hearing aid — but paid for it myself. Not hearing was not an option for me, so I was willing to do whatever was necessary.

> With free-flowing, nonstop tears, I at least had the presence of mind to realize that a cochlear implant was my next step.

With much confidence, I eagerly awaited the day of my initial stimulation. One by one, my threshold and comfort levels for each electrode were determined. Then, with great anticipation, all my electrodes were turned on and I fully expected to understand speech once again. Instead, I heard nothing but static. I became inconsolable. Again, I cried and internal hysteria resumed. There was no way I was ever going to make sense of those electrical impulses, especially not at the age of 50.

Immediately after the initial stimulation process, I flew to New York for the annual seders my mother prepared every Passover. My son, my brother, and my cousins were all there to witness how well I was doing with my newly found hearing. I put up as strong a face as I could, but during those moments of solitude with my immediate family, they saw through the false bravado. Despite my valiant attempts to practice listening to speech on audiotapes, I was in deep emotional agony.

Two weeks later, I returned to the cochlear implant center for the second programming of my implant — and, this time, the programming seemed to work. Suddenly, I could understand speech! Later that day, I happily spoke with my parents by telephone. Not with quite the same ease as my hearing aid, but I understood them, nevertheless. And, I was grateful for every crumb! I noticed that the 24-hour roaring in my head had finally subsided and I could sleep. However, not being experienced in surgical recuperation, I thought my postoperative pain was normal — even when it continued unabated for the next few months.

Within six months, it looked like I was growing another earlobe — a rather reddened one, in fact — and the pain became so unbearable that I couldn't use my processor for more than an hour at a time. The surgeon prescribed steroid pills, but they did not seem to have any effect. He then suggested that we explant the internal portion of the device because he felt that was what was causing the problems. He further recommended that I implant my other ear, the one I had unsuccessfully tried to aid on Helen Beebe's advice so many years ago. My surgeon believed I could learn to understand speech as easily with my right ear since listening was a "brain thing." Moreover, he felt I should implant my other ear with a different manufacturer's device (though not with its latest generation) in order to minimize all potential problems.

So, my mother and I traipsed into the doctor's office, ready to have him again check me into the hospital. When he looked at my "second earlobe," he said it seemed to have subsided and become less red; he recommended canceling the explantation, so I did. Three more months passed and the pain became truly excruciating even when I wasn't using the processor. This time, I consulted a pediatric cochlear implant surgeon who immediately began treating me for a *staphylococcus aureus* infection, placing me on IV antibiotics at home three times a day for three weeks. The angry redness soon dissipated and the size of my second earlobe became quite small, but my skin flap had ruptured and the internal stimulator was extruded. There was no choice now but to schedule an emergency explantation.

At this point, I consulted with a third cochlear implant surgeon, who argued against using a different device. Like the second surgeon, he insisted that my problem was a staph infection that I likely contracted during surgery. Quick decisions had to be made and, in consideration of my financial interests as well as my abject fear of living in a silent world, I followed the first surgeon's advice and chose implantation of a different device with an older model in the right ear. This decision proved to be costlier than I imagined.

I had three more weeks of massive IV antibiotic treatments at home to finally rid myself of the staph infection. I then made arrangements to have my second implant surgery performed by the third surgeon I had consulted. The problem with the second surgery was not that a different manufacturer's device was implanted; it was my right ear. A whole year transpired before I was even able to understand a few common everyday expressions. Rendered powerless, I had to depend on faxes and other people telling me what the other party was saying on the telephone. That I had to rely on others was detestably out of character for me. I grieved all that year; fury and depression reigned.

> A whole year transpired before I was even able to understand a few common expressions. I grieved all that year; fury reigned.

By then, I had no faith in any one doctor and consequently consulted with two more cochlear implant surgeons on my future status as a hearing person. Eleven months after my second surgery, three doctors agreed that I should reimplant my left ear since they observed no signs of a staph infection. I was determined to rise again; my hopes for a salvageable future were pinned on this. On the day of my third surgery, my brother was there to hold my hand and bring me home. He saw my pain and the beginning of my vertigo, which stayed with me for weeks, along with bouts of vomiting that accompanied each of my frequent and severe episodes of dizziness.

When I was programmed to hear with my third processor, I could again finally understand speech! I spoke to my mother on the telephone, and as she conveyed this to my dying father, he shed his last tears of muted gladness. It was just two weeks later that he passed away.

I tried comparing hearing aid usage to cochlear implant usage, but found it was like comparing apples to oranges. With my hearing aid, I had a severe hearing loss; with my implant, I have a profound loss. The two are incomparable. Without question, and for many reasons, I prefer hearing with my hearing aid to hearing with the cochlear implant. Yet I continue to be grateful for my implant even though surgeries on both ears caused me to become totally deaf. The surgeries eliminated the small amount of residual hearing I had left in each ear, which means I will no longer be able to take advantage of any improved hearing aid technology in the future. For now, I'm still able to use the phone and to understand most of what I hear, just not as easily as before.

My episodic vertigo continues today. Just as there's a very small chance of getting a staph infection from surgery and an even smaller chance of having it medically mismanaged, there's also a very small chance of one's balance system becoming permanently impaired as a result of the surgery. I seem to have been a victim of the odds in all three cases. To say that I am extremely shy of further surgeries would be putting it mildly.

> The yawning abyss of silence angers and frightens me. Therefore, I've become even more stridently vocal about the A-V way of life.

The transition to profound deafness has changed me more than anything. I continue to do without listening systems while making it my business to always sit in the front row when listening to speakers. Although I still think of myself as a functionally hearing person, primarily defined by my large city ethnic roots, I'm fully aware of the fact that, but for the cochlear implant, I continually stand on the precipice of total deafness. The yawning abyss of silence both angers and frightens me. Therefore, I've become even more stridently vocal about the A-V way of life and the need for binaural hearing.

I've become more cynical about issues concerning calculating friendships, inherent biases, stereotypes, labels, and historical revisionists. I don't like it when professional colleagues say to me, "You speak so well," with *for a deaf person* remaining the unspoken and unfinished thought, or "I met with Ellen before and tried to discuss issues with her. I'm not sure there's much listening going on. Maybe that's the hearing loss."

Similarly, I dislike when people with hearing loss are objectified; professional organizations that serve "the deaf and hard of hearing" need to rethink their

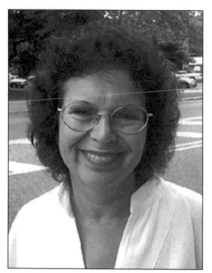

I recently purchased a BTE processor for the implant in my right ear. Although my motivation is not especially high at this stage of my life, what remains to be seen is whether understanding speech through that ear is possible after a lifetime of dormancy.

own semantics. Before I lost my residual hearing, I would have held my tongue. Now, I speak (and write) my mind. I'm weary of pejorative labels and stereotypic notions, and I find low expectations even less tolerable when emanating from those who supposedly embrace the Auditory-Verbal philosophy. I no longer endure condescension in muted tones. On the contrary, I rage against silent and misguided voices.

Philosophical Reflections

My father taught me well. He taught me always to look for the silver lining in every cloud. Indeed, I feel fortunate that I have loved my primary career choice as an Auditory-Verbal professional. Working with families has been most rewarding of all. Each time I am with grieving parents, I feel their sorrow, weep again, and am glad that I can ease their pain. I feel as though I have accomplished much — establishing three A-V programs and helping many professionals who, in turn, have helped many more parents and their children. I know I've made a difference in the field of deafness, and this is immensely satisfying to me.

For the past six years, I have mentored professionals who aspire to become certified A-V therapists. I have conducted A-V training workshops, made professional presentations, consulted with families via week-long home visits, and written a variety of articles and research papers. While traveling around the world, I have met wonderful parents who have taken the A-V route without weekly professional assistance. I have also met many professionals who want to learn about the unlimited possibilities of A-V therapy, and I have relished the freedom to do this work. My choices and time are mine.

I recently purchased a BTE processor for the implant in my right ear. It seemed the right time to do this because I had to put my money where my mouth was and start learning how to listen in a 58-year-old unused ear. Although my motivation is not especially high at this stage of my life, what remains to be seen is whether understanding speech through that ear is possible after a lifetime of dormancy. Perhaps if I am indeed able to attain at least 50% comprehension of speech in my right ear (certainly not as good as the 80% in my left ear, but a lot better than the 10% now in the right), then I will not harbor such great fear that the device in my left ear might fail me one day.

My very independent son is quite open about my deafness and my trials with various hearing prostheses. Since he was a toddler, he has intuitively understood my need for relatively quiet environments and good lighting in dark places. I daresay he knows more than the average person about surgical risks. He fully understands the implications of the genetics of deafness on any children he might have one day, and he knows the value of hearing. Although unquestionably sensitive to hearing issues, he demonstrates his impatience with me, too. Those times typically have nothing to do with my hearing loss. As an only child raised by a single mother, we continue to have a close relationship even though he lives in Atlanta and I reside in Fort Lauderdale, Florida.

My brother, now a bank executive and still a hearing aid user, will always be my compatriot in deafness. We speak on the telephone almost daily. He continues to be a good sounding board. My brother, my son, and I continue to travel together occasionally, since our love for exotic places represents a common interest.

My significant other, who has loved me unconditionally for the past 20 years, still does not quite understand all the ramifications of deafness. On a simplistic level, he knows I cannot carry a tune and that I hear nothing when I sleep or shower. But how can he truly know what I go through when he understands speech so effortlessly, sings so beautifully, loves music, and the telephone is his most important business tool? He accepts me for who I am and all the hearing paraphernalia (i.e., battery charger, hearing prosthesis dehumidifier, rechargeable batteries, cochlear implant processor spare parts) that must accompany me wherever I go.

I've learned that life can turn any direction in a second. Although a hearing loss has always been a part of me, it has created some unexpected and unwanted detours in my life. I don't believe it has made me a better person; being a Pollyanna about a sensory disability is not my way of thinking. If anything, I feel that limited hearing has hindered me instead. I am not one who feels that goodness comes out of deafness, that deafness gave me a purpose in life, that I am special because of deafness, or that I was given deafness because some higher being felt I could handle it. Goodness needs no baggage. For me, deafness is a condition that merely intensifies awareness of what I am.

Sometimes, the greater the deafness the easier it is to learn wrong lessons from it. Truth turns into myth, mortals into heroes, luck into fate, and fears into badges. As my brother always said: "I've no choice but to play the cards dealt me." And, I feel that I've done a pretty good job of defeating the enemy. At least I've won more than I've lost. Yet, if I or any member of my family were presented a "do-over" opportunity, we would banish deafness forever. In recurrent dreams, I hear without a device while swimming naked in pools and oceans. What unbridled joy it must be!

Advice for Parents

In conclusion, I offer the following advice for parents:

- ❧ Choose your words wisely. Know that they affect stereotypes and expectations, including your child's self-concept. If you want an A-V child, then believe that you will enable your child to become a hearing person. No, your child will never have normal hearing, but he or she can still become a functionally hearing individual.
- ❧ A hearing device is the most important thing your child owns. Give it the care it needs. From the moment your child obtains this device, it must be worn during all waking hours.

- Believe in yourself. You can enable your child to become a hearing and speaking child despite deafness, even if you don't have access to a local A-V professional. Seek support only from those who share your vision.
- Bathe your child in natural melodic spoken language. Talk to your child about what he sees and does. Explain everything about everything.
- Teach your child how to behave. Do not let the hearing impairment affect your management of his behaviors.
- Make sure your child is well-rounded. Provide as many experiences as possible in sports, music, arts and crafts, and so forth, and permit your child to develop a special interest.
- Say what you mean and mean what you say. Be forthright and direct with your child. Communicate what you want and need, and how you feel.
- Instill a love of reading. Read to your child. Let your child see you read newspapers, books, and magazines. Supply reading materials of any kind.
- Relinquish ownership of the deafness. Begin transferring it to your child as soon as language is understood and used like that of a typical 4-year-old with normal hearing who is considered linguistically competent.
- Let your child fail. Let him learn from his mistakes and learn how to deal with difficult situations. Give him tools so he can learn how to learn and therefore become independent.
- Teach your child to laugh at himself. See the humor in pathos. Be sure your child understands that what we do and say can put others at ease about his hearing loss. Be sure that your child knows no one is perfect and that everyone feels some insecurity. Help him learn to confront his own weaknesses and accept them for what they are.
- Think things through. Use common sense and be logical when explaining things to an older child. Appeal to his sense of reason so he understands the pros and cons of any situation.
- Teach your child to be a *mensch*. Model what a decent, upright, mature, and responsible person does. In giving examples, tell him what you're going to tell him, then tell him, and tell him again what you told him. It will eventually sink in, even with teenagers.
- Practice what you preach. If you don't want others to stereotype or apply pejorative labels to your child or his hearing differences, then don't apply them to others, regardless of race, ethnicity, religious, or sexual orientation. Embrace diversity.
- Buy the best hearing device possible.
- Behave yourself.
- Be honest.
- Sing, laugh, and enjoy life.

ABOUT THE EDITOR

Warren Estabrooks, M.Ed., Dip. Ed. Deaf, Cert. AVT®

WARREN ESTABROOKS IS DIRECTOR OF THE AUDITORY LEARNING CENTRE at the Learning to Listen Foundation (LTLF), Toronto, Canada. Mr. Estabrooks is a global consultant who lectures worldwide on Auditory-Verbal therapy, auditory (re)habilitation, auditory learning, childhood hearing impairment, and cochlear implant habilitation. He is instrumental in worldwide training and development of professionals in related pediatric and adult disciplines.

Mr. Estabrooks is a lifetime member and the International Ambassador of the Alexander Graham Bell Association for the Deaf and Hard of Hearing. He is registered with the College of Teachers of Ontario and has held the position of assistant professor at the University of Toronto, Faculty of Medicine. His professional honors include the Susann Schmid-Giovannini Award for International Excellence in Auditory-Verbal Practice, the Professional of the Year Award from the International Organization for the Education of the Hearing Impaired (INPROSEC), the Dr. E.W. Wight Memorial Scholarship, and the Peter R. Newman Humanitarian Award in recognition of his contribution to children who are deaf and their families around the world. He has been acclaimed to the Canadian Who's Who (2005) as a Canadian of influence.

The Learning to Listen Foundation received the first International Voice of Deafness Award (2003) for a program, and the Auditory Learning Centre (LTLF) was twice honored as the International Program of the Year by INPROSEC.

Mr. Estabrooks has made significant contributions to the literature, including *Do You Hear That?* (1992), *Hear & Listen! Talk & Sing!* (1994), *Auditory-Verbal Therapy for Parents and Professionals* (1994), *The ABC's of AVT* (1995), *Cochlear Implants for Kids* (1998), *The Baby Is Listening* (2000), *50 FAQs About AVT (50 Frequently Asked Questions About Auditory-Verbal Therapy)* (2001), *Songs for Listening! Songs for Life!* (2003), *The Six-Sound Song* (2003), *Listen to This! Volume I* (2004), and *Auditory-Verbal Therapy and Practice* (2005).